The Green

Jamie Kershaw

chipmunkapublishing
the mental health publisher

All rights reserved, no part of this publication may be reproduced by any means, electronic, mechanical photocopying, documentary, film or in any other format without prior written permission of the publisher.

>Published by
>Chipmunkapublishing
>PO Box 6872
>Brentwood
>Essex CM13 1ZT
>United Kingdom

http://www.chipmunkapublishing.com

Copyright © Jamie Kershaw 2011

Edited by D B Kershaw

Chipmunkapublishing gratefully acknowledge the support of Arts Council England.

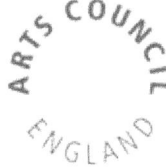

One Third of people with schizophrenia recover fully; One Third will have another episode; and One Third will get on as normal with occasional intermittent symptoms.

-Rosenberg

Jamie Kershaw

Author Biography

Jamie was born in 1978 in York, N Yorks, and currently lives in Scarborough. He was educated at Hull University, E Yorks, 2002-2007, during which time he completed numerous half marathons, 10kms and the Paris Marathon in April 2006 in 3 hrs 25 mins (in response to brother Chris's New York marathon 2000 in 3hrs 37 mins!) He has also bungee jumped, white-water rafted, and firewalked. He attended Durham School 1992-97.

However, in September 1998 he was diagnosed with schizophrenia aged 20, and over a ten year period has had several hospital admissions mainly in Cross Lane Hospital, Scarborough, and St Luke's Hospital, Middlesborough. These experiences are detailed in subsequent chapters.

The script for *The Green Dragon* was written over a two year period in Scarborough whilst living with family, and is his second book. As it is an autobiography, *The Green Dragon* is non-fiction.

He is something of an amateur musician and pianist, occasionally playing a live gig - also playing basic guitar, harmonica, and viola. Whilst at university he spent one year in Canada on an exchange based at Dalhousie University, Halifax, Nova Scotia. He has travelled somewhat across Canada and through various countries of Europe.

There are thoughts of writing a sequel to his first fiction book, *Plan 103f*, as well as writing a non-fiction music book, a children's book, and a book about Scarborough.

Jamie Kershaw

Acknowledgements

Dedicated to Christina and the boys

With thanks to Mum and Dad for being there always

"The innocent and the beautiful have no enemy but time"
(W B Yeats 1856-1939)

Jamie Kershaw

The Green Dragon

Prologue

One July night in 2006, I was on the run. I had covered 15 miles on foot already by this point on the roads, and was almost at the village of Sheriff Hutton, North Yorkshire. Suddenly a police van passed, drove on, turned round and came up behind me as I ran. Upon being requested to pull over I declined the request and continued moving at a pace. The police van continued to follow me closely, up the hill and into the village itself. Suddenly at the junction a second police van had been summoned to cut me off and pulled out in front of me. I dodged through. Then the vans did a manoeuvre to cut me off again, I dashed between the wall and the van and just got through the gap.

Further down the road an officer was waiting brandishing a truncheon, telling me to pull over by the van. I did an impromptu rugby dummy pass/shimmy move and the two of us had a chase, only there was suddenly a German Shepherd on my tail too. "Kill him, Barney!" they yelled at the dog. Somehow the dog decided to run alongside me for a while without jumping up, pulling me down, and tearing me to pieces.

My only means of escape came suddenly - a tiny gap in the hedge; now or never as I ran, so I nipped through, onto the castle playing fields in the dark. It worked. They were thrown off my tail. Without too much ado I climbed the fence, cut across country and à la Boyz in the Hood, secretly cut across some back gardens away from the chase. After some time I heard a noise in the sky and saw a searchlight approaching. They had called a helicopter over to look for me. I hid in the hedgerow and gradually made for the woods. Here I decided to avoid the police trap and double back on myself.

24 hours later I was knocking on my brother's door in York. I had made it 30 miles to York, cross country, on foot. Fields, woodland, streams, hedgerows; I felt quite literally dragged backwards through the gorse bushes by the time I arrived;

sleepless, cold, hungry and exhausted. He ain't heavy, he's my brother! This, however, was only the beginning…

World Events 1978–2011

- 1978 Queen Elizabeth II on the throne: an Elizabethan Age
- James Callaghan (Labour) Prime Minister: (1976-79)
- The Winter of Discontent 1979
His autobiography "Time and Chance" published 1987
- The Author was born, 1978
- 1979 Egypt-Israel Peace Treaty
- The taking of US hostages in Iran
- A Soviet invasion of Afghanistan
- Jimmy Carter (Democrat) 39th US President (1977-81)
- UN Secretary General Kurt Waldheim (Austria) (1971-81)
- 1976-84 Bjorn Borg v John McEnroe (Wimbledon Men's Tennis)
- 1978-90 Martina Navratilova (Wimbledon Ladies Tennis)
- 1979 Margaret Thatcher (Conservative) Prime Minister: (1979-90)
Thatcherism, Privatisation, "The Downing Street Years" autobiography 1993
- 1980 Moscow Olympic Games
- 1981 Prince Charles married Princess Diana
- 1984 Los Angeles Olympic Games
- 1986 Chernobyl nuclear leakage
- Ronald Reagan (Republican) 40th US President (1981-89)
- Music of the 1980's: Nick Kershaw, Spandau Ballet, Whitesnake, Queen, Elton John, Soft Cell, Stone Roses, Tpau, Michael Jackson, Madonna, Petshop Boys, A-Ha, Wham, Dire Straits, Bananarama, Salt 'n' Peppa, ABBA, Def Leppard, Metallica, Aerosmith, INXS, U2, Richard Marx, Meatloaf, Guns 'n' Roses, Men at Work, Michael Bolton…
- 1985 Boris Becker youngest ever Wimbledon winner
- Exxon Valdez Oil spillage Alaska
- UN Secretary General Javier Perez de Cuellar (Peru) (1982-92)
- Mikael Gorbachev Soviet President (1985-95)
Perestroika, Glasnost, Abolition of Communism, Dissolution of Soviet Union 1991
- Steffi Graff (Wimbledon Ladies Tennis 1988-96)

- 1988 Seoul Olympic Games
- 1989 The Falkland Islands War
- 1989 Tiananmen Square protests and massacre
- 1989 East and West Germany reunited (Berlin Wall fell)
- George H W Bush (Republican) 41st US President (1989-92)
- John Major (Conservative) Prime Minister: (1990-97)
- UN Secretary General Boutros Boutros Ghali (Egypt) (1992-97)
- William Jefferson Clinton (Democrat) 42nd US President (1992-2000)
"Giving" his Autobiography published 2008
- 1991 Gulf War – United Nations invaded Iraq following Iraq invading Kuwait 1990
- 1992 Barcelona Olympic Games
- 1992 Annus Horribilis (Queen Elizabeth II)
- 1992 Andre Agassi wins Wimbledon
- 1993 US National Health Care Programme
- 1994 Channel Tunnel opened; The 'Chunnel'
- 1994 Haiti Crisis and Rwandan Genocide
- Boris Yeltsin Russian President 1991-2000
- 1992-95 War in Bosnia and Herzegovina
- 1993-2000 Pete Sampras (Wimbledon Men's Tennis)
- 1996 Atlanta Olympic Games
- 1997 Princess Diana died in car crash in Paris
- 1998 Hurricane Katrina flattened New Orleans
- Music of the 1990's: Oasis, Pulp, Blur, Radiohead, Portishead, Crowded House, R.E.M, The Cranberries, The Orb, Bryan Adams, Take That, Boyzone, Westlife, Michael Jackson, Madonna, Elton John, Guns n Roses, U2, The Spice Girls, Atomic Kitten, D:Ream, Haddaway, Jamiroquai…
- Tony Blair (New Labour) Prime Minister: (1997-2008)
- UN Secretary General Koffi Annan (Ghana) (1997-2008)
- 2000 Sydney Olympic Games
- 2000 George W Bush (Republican) 43rd US President (2000-2008)
John Kerry and Al Gore (An Inconvenient Truth 2008) were both defeated by Bush
- Vladimir Putin elected Russian Federation President (2000-)

- 2000-2011 Venus and Serena Williams (Ladies Wimbledon Tennis)
- 2002-2011 Roger Federer (Men's Wimbledon Tennis)
- 2001 '9/11' New York Twin Towers destroyed by Al-Qaeda Terrorists
- 2003 Invasion of Iraq and Afghanistan
- 2003 England won the Rugby World Cup (Jonny Wilkinson)
- December, 2004 Malaysian Tsunami
- 2004 Athens Olympic Games
- July, 2005 London bombings
- 2006 Saddam Hussein (Iraqi President) Hanged, Alexander Litvinyenko (KGB) poisoned
- 2007 Benazir Bhutto assassinated (Pakistani Prime Minister)
- 2008 Beijing Olympic Games
- Gordon Brown (Labour) Prime Minister: (2008-10)
- UN Secretary General Ban Ki Moon (Korea) (2008-)
- Barack Obama (Democrat) 44th US President (2008-) first Black President.
Hillary Clinton US Secretary of State (Would have been first female President)
- 2009 Deaths of Luciano Pavarotti (Opera star), Michael Jackson (King of Pop), Stephen Gately (Boyzone), Patrick Swayze (Film Star)
- 2011 Egypt Liberated (President Mubarak brought down)
- Libya defending Colonel Gadaffi
- Music of the 21st Century: Sugababes, Girls Aloud, JLS, The Saturdays, Pink, Adele, John Legend, Seal, Duffy, Madonna, Elton John, Michael Jackson, One Night Only, Jay-Z, Blue, Beyoncé, Westlife, Take That (reformed), Coldplay, Snow Patrol, Paulo Nuttini, Robbie Williams, Kate Perry, Lady GaGa, Lilly Allen, Olly Murs, Matt Cardel, Jamie Archer, Joe McElderry, Will Young, Gareth Gates, Leona Lewis, LeMarr, Alexandra Burke, Journey South…
- 2011 Japanese nuclear leakage
- 29th April 2011 The Royal Wedding: Prince William married Kate Middleton
- May 2011 Osama Bin Laden executed
- 2012 London Olympic Games

Jamie Kershaw

Chapter One
The Early Years

When I was born the name given on the York maternity hospital card, UK, read 'baby of Jean Kershaw'. Mum kept detailed notes of my first seven years, with photographs. Quoting from these notes I know that I checked in at 12.05pm September 27th, 1978. I weighed 8lb 13oz and was administered with 1mg Konakion. Mum and Dad decided on 'James Alexander' before long, though. We lived in a small Yorkshire 'double'-village called Beadlam/Nawton, where mum and dad still live today in 2011.

For three and a half months I was breast-fed, and sometimes required six or seven feeds a night. My first smile was at three weeks old, grinning at my dad. At four and a half months I was bottle-fed, even being given some brandy to pacify me. We had a neighbour called Rene Keast who would help babysit, and she has remained "part of the family" all my life. I understood phrases like "Where is Christopher?", and at six months had my first visit to Spain.

Mum had me bottle-fed on cow's milk until the eczema came, then I was given goat's milk, which worked fine. At eight months I was given a taste of antibiotics. My first teeth came at eight and a half months. I would often chuckle at the other children's antics whom I met. I was given a turquoise 'blankie' which accompanied me for about eight years.

We had two goldfish, Toby and Sam. The first time I stood unaided was at nine months, and I used to wave dad off in the morning as he went to work. At 10 months I developed bad eczema and was on a non-bovine diet. I walked across the kitchen unaided at one year old.

First words included "Wot's dat?" at 17 months, and I was fascinated by animals, saying things like "Dat's a duck…water". In the street I got on with other boys, and when I heard music I would conduct with raised index fingers. At 2 years I would say

"Are you busy, mum?", and "Have you gone upstairs, Jonny?". At three I could count to ten and recite nursery rhymes, such as "Old king coalman", "Wasn't that a dirty dish?" and "after later." I liked broccoli and green vegetables, apparently. At three I was given a hand-puppet monkey whom I named 'Mongrish'. He accompanied me for many years.

My first real memories are of Spain, the Casita and my Grandparents' villa. We used to go on holiday there in the summer and Christmas holidays, and I can still recall the aeroplane flying high above the clouds, and wanting to reach out to touch them. We flew to Alicante airport on the East coast of Spain where my granddad (mum's father) would be there waiting in the car, having helped with the travel costs. Mum, Dad, Chris, Jonny and I were the luckiest lot in the world to be going there. Chris was the eldest of us three brothers, Jonny the middle, and I the youngest, being only three years of age when we went for the last time.

One of these earliest memories is of my mother jumping into a swimming pool with a dress on to stop me drowning. My armbands had sprung a leak and everyone else just watched the whole thing from their sunbeds. Also, at a Benidorm beach, a wild cat was prowling round and eventually pounced on Chris's chicken dinner and stole it from his hands as he was about to take a bite. I remember finding a lizard in the bedroom and Jonny discovering that a lizard's tail actually drops off when grabbed, in self-defence. At that time Jonny would also refer to the oranges on the trees as 'little whoppers'.

My three other earliest memories of Spain are the strawberries and cream that grandma provided; a trip up a mountain to a honey farm where a swarm of bees produced a variety of honey which could be sampled for free. Also, from the age of three I remember Christmas. One Christmas eve I was put to bed early while the 'older' people stayed up to wrap presents. Unsurprisingly I was unable to sleep that night.

Back on home turf, the very first school I ever attended was a local nursery at Nunnington on a farm of sorts. I have been told that, there, I was something of a monster by the age of five – pushing, biting, and sabotaging others, but don't believe a word of it! I was good at puzzles, and loved stories and being sung to. At five years I developed whooping cough, and read 'The Wind in the Willows' and 'Famous 5'.

After a short time at Nunnington nursery school I went to Nawton County Primary School until the age of seven. In the morning my first words would be, "Am I going to school today?"

In the summer of '83 I learnt to ride a bike. Then also in 1983 I was told not to watch 'Jaws' with my older brothers, and not to go to the disco across the road until I was older, at which point I pushed my plate across the table and shouted, "You don't let me do anything – I wish I was six!" Two hours later mum found me in the disco.

At six years I developed asthma and was given becotide and ventolin inhalers, and also suffered from allergies to mown grass and horse hair. I said things like "Girls smell of stew", and "Girls get on my neck", and at seven years I had gone off girls altogether, preferring to swim at Ampleforth and ride horses at Sinnington. Mum started to teach me piano at six years, and got me onto viola with Jill Bowman, and recorder with school, for all of which I displayed some aptitude. Around this age my brothers and I were given a pair of boxing gloves and I once gave Jonny a black eye in a bout. Another time, Chris and I were messing round in the back garden and I must have found a stick somewhere, because he keeps reminding me that I hit him on the nose with it, causing a bleed. He came after me soon afterwards!

Primary School was a ten minute walk from home. Somedays I would be home for dinner, other times I stayed at school. There were things going on – school yard squabbles, groups and gangs, games of 'British Bulldogs' and 'Red Rover'. I can recall the

Halkon brothers, James and Ben, and the Foots brothers Alec, Barry, Trevor and Brian. Also Joanna Robinson (the first girl I ever kissed), Darren, Paul, Mike Scott, Kit Brown, Kevin Prendergast, Ginny Leonard, Jake Leonard, and Paul Featherstone, who once started a fight with me in the field on the way back home. He told me to take a swing for him so I did then he responded. Apparently Steve Mackley saw the whole thing from his home down the hill in the street, he told me later.

James Halkon was gang leader on account of being brought up on a farm. He was tough. The shed on the farm was used as HQ. However, my membership of this gang was pretty short-lived and I can't remember the details now. Once, on the farm, James, Ben and myself were messing round on top of a stack of hay bales and eventually we decided to climb down. As my foot went for the ladder I slipped and fell to the hay-sheep-shit-covered concrete floor and blacked out for a while. Ben and James both found this amusing. Funny my arse!

Another time I had cycled up the lane to the farm and James beckoned me to the local skip where there were great piles of leaves, mattresses, disused cabinets and other rubbish. In a nutshell, we set fire to a small pile of leaves and it ended up setting the entire tip on fire. We ran back to the farm shouting, "The tip's on fire! It wasn't us!" I was sent home on my bike and James was no doubt given a ticking off, too. The last time I saw James Halkon was in the 'Feathers' pub in Helmsley in 1998. We hadn't much to say to each other any more, though.

Kevin Prendergast used to show off a karate black belt at the age of seven. We were never too sure if it was for real or 'acquired' by other means.

Mike Scott was a judo expert from an early age and once demonstrated a spectacular throw to his friends. Only I was the target. He flipped me over his shoulder with ease and I crashed to the ground, flat on my back. When I left Nawton Primary School, the next time I saw Mike was as a sixteen year old. He was dating Catriona Begg, also from Beadlam/Nawton. I went to see them with my French exchange colleague Thomas Lefranc for an hour. About a year later our neighbour Rene Keast told us the news that Mike had collapsed while playing basketball and died. He was just seventeen. I attended the funeral and recognised several people there of whom there were many. His older brother Ben had known me during a summer job at the Pheasant Inn, Harome. His family set up a charity in Mike's memory – Cardiac Risk in the Young (C.R.Y.). I was affected badly by Mike's death and once drove to the graveyard on my own on a dark evening and attempted to resurrect him by singing and shouting to him to get up again. I swear that his spirit came to me that night, I felt an otherwise inexplicable emotion that night. I never knew how to handle this. I thought it best to give the family space and never really came to terms with Mike's death.

Back to Primary school days, Barry Foots also had a September birthday and our birthday parties occurred at similar times. Once at Barry's party I was challenged to a fight with somebody with whom I had no intention of fighting. Somehow the situation diluted itself and I got off lightly. The Foots boys had built the world's best tree-house in their garden and all the kids loved to climb up to it. The eldest, Alec, once bunked off school and hid in the tree house. That was talked about for weeks. Around the age of seven, I did look forwards to Junior Club for which the entry requirement was to be seven years old. This would involve gym games, bike rides and swimming sessions at Ryedale school pool.

My worst nightmare at this age was probably with Nicky Brown, who lived just two doors away up our street. His antics ranged from shoving ants down my back to making me swallow worms, chilli peppers, and chasing me down the street with a tennis racket. His dad Ernest used to breed puppy dogs and once invited me to see them but my dad wouldn't let me keep a dog. These troubles ceased when I went to boarding school, and a new world began.

Our back garden was popular for birthdays. Mum and Dad bought us a miniature roller-coaster which lasted for years. Dad taught us how to ride a bike in the street progressing from three wheels to two. They also bought us a water slide. Half the village turned up one summer's day to slide along the water slide, belly up. Mark and Robin Rymer, Steve Mackley, Andy, Paul and Richard Edwards, the Foots and others. The lawn ended up soggy, and was written off for a while, but it was all worth it.

Mum once made a homemade chocolate birthday cake in the shape of a train. The cake had Cadbury fingers and Wagon wheels for the wheels. I can still recall that.

Another of my Primary school memories is of Ginny Leonard. She once came to the house to see me and opened a little red satchel to reveal her bra collection of which she seemed proud! I wasn't sure where to look. Nor was I convinced that she required such items at that age.

At school we had an annual sports day and my first ever accolade was gained here. I came second in a fifty yard dash and was presented with a token ribbon. James Halkon won and Barry Foots came third. The longer race of a complete lap at that age seemed an absolute mile. Little did I realise my later interests would be in this area. We learnt basic ball skills at Nawton Primary in the school yard and there was a good climbing frame facility in the field as well. Once, I played piano in front of the whole school –a short piece by Haydn.

Mrs Downie taught Maths and English and used to make sure that I took my inhaler whenever I needed it. I suffered from asthma as a child. I can remember my Dad's mum – Bradford Nana – walking me to school on occasion quite proudly. Mum comes from the Midlands/Nottingham and Dad from Bradford. When we used to visit Bradford Nana and Grandpa, we always drove the same route, stopping at Carrefour supermarket for groceries and lunch in the café on the way. Dad drove fast over the bumpy bits which made us laugh in the back of the car. On

The Green Dragon

reaching Bradford we parked further up the road and ran to the house at 308 Kings Road. The next door neighbour's Rough Collie called Sandy always barked at us. Nana usually made a salad tea and homemade macaroons. Grandpa Billy played dominoes and tiddlywinks with us, or played us some guitar at which he was very adept. His garden shed was my "boat", my cockpit – the vice was a steering wheel, while the cables, rakes, spades and forks all served an equally important purpose in the "boat". When we left the house to drive home, Nana always gave each of us boys £1 to take with us. She always kept a ready supply of blackcurrant throat lozenges in the cupboard. Nana always kept my dad supplied with blue mint rock for his car. He kept this in a special jam jar in the glove compartment and offered it round before we set off.

Also, on our trips to Bradford we used to visit Aunty Jean and cousin Jonty. For many years they also lived with Uncle Frank, Jonty's dad. After some time, for whatever reasons, Jean and Frank's relationship fell apart so they divorced and Aunty Jean moved house with Jonty to the Eccleshill area of Bradford where Jonty still lives to this day. For a while Aunty Jean took up jogging. She was known as 'kid' by my dad (her brother), and would always lay on a huge spread for us all at her house when we visited. However, in her latter years the doctors diagnosed her with a type of cancer, and sadly, after a long time, she died, leaving Jonty with the house. Jonty tried to teach us some basic 'blues guitar', and owned a fine military collection in his attic, particularly enjoying painting model soldiers and arranging them into ranks. I will talk more of Jonty in chapter ten, 'Family'. Uncle Frank sadly passed away on 13th April 2011 after a long struggle. Jonty and his sister Jenny were in charge of funeral arrangements in Beverley, and Jonty made a tribute to his dad for everybody. I attended with mum and dad.

One time at home, when I was four, mum and dad had bought some alphabet fridge magnets and I was playing with various letters. Suddenly I spelt out the word 'Morew'. Dad asked me what it meant, and I told him suddenly, "Ger out lad, your house is on fire!" They never let me forget about that one! Jonny and

Chris were both amused, as well. Jonny was into motorbikes from an early age and owned a 90cc Kawasaki which we rode up the Howl woods and on the disused airfield at Wombleton. I crashed once whilst giving Steve Mackley a lift down the Howl track. It put me off. I never got 'back on the horse' and nobody told me to. Two other instances of not 'getting back on the horse' were literally being thrown off a horse at the Bowmans' house in Gilling into a patch of nettles, and then whilst sailing at Ripon Sailing Club with mum – we capsized in a freak gust of wind which blew over every boat on the lake. I ended up swimming to shore whilst mum waited with the boat for the life boat to pick her up. I remember the water being not too cold at the time.

Whilst at Nawton Primary School I began to learn to swim, using the swimming pools at Ryedale school with Junior Club, and at Ampleforth College where my parents taught music, as well as learning to canoe and attend hand-eye ball skills courses. In 1985, aged 7, I ran three miles for 'Live Aid'. Running all over the world, I like it! I like it! You get the picture. Bob Geldof in his prime, Genesis and Phil Collins etc. If only I had understood the actual concept of Live Aid it would have been a far greater experience!

One summer's day, Dad had invited me to come and listen to his school talk on Esperanto at Terrington Hall. I wasn't yet at the school, though it wasn't long before one sunny afternoon at home, mum and dad asked me, "Would you like to go to boarding school?" Without knowing anything about it I replied that I would like to go, and quite emphatically at that. That school was to be Terrington Hall Preparatory School where I would spend the next five years of my life as a 'sponsored pupil'. An extremely generous and anonymous old boy had decided to sponsor a pupil throughout his time at school, and that lucky person was me. My eighth birthday happened within a month of my starting at Terrington, and that is what follows.

Why I hadn't chosen Ryedale school just down the road, like everyone else, or Ampleforth, where mum and dad both taught,

I'm not sure. But who cares! Jonny and Chris both had the same schooling route via Ampleforth College and York Sixth Form College, but I was different.

A month before my eighth birthday in September 1987, I went to boarding school. I didn't realise it then, but for the next ten years I would be at boarding school. The first was to be Terrington Hall Preparatory School in North Yorkshire. The then Headmaster, Desmond Gray, and his wife Gill (Headmatron) made us all feel welcome and helped get us into uniform before the school year started. Mum and Dad were already music teachers at the school as well as Ampleforth, and had been offered sponsorship for my place at the school. My entire five years at Terrington were on an anonymously assisted place. The sponsor to this day has refused to be identified so I have never been able to express my gratitude or whatever else I might want to express.

The first contact I had with a fellow Terringtonian was a postcard from Bonner Earl saying that he would be my mentor-friend whilst I found my feet. We were the same age and in the same year. I started in form two, having been at Nawton, instead of form one. There were six forms – one to six - with one being the youngest and six being mainly twelve-year-olds. I spent five years there, and each form was divided into an (a) and a (b) depending on how bright the pupil proved to be.

Comments from my first ever school report at Terrington included in Science: "Jamie has worked willingly and hard throughout the term and he is just beginning to come out of his shell and show some character," (Tim Chapman). On viola "Jamie is a very promising young musician. He produces a good sound on his viola and the basics of his technique have been well founded. I enjoy our lessons together immensely and hope he does too," (C A Johnson). Five years later I was awarded a music exhibition to go on to Durham school, owing to playing piano, and viola, and singing.

The Headmaster's first school report for me in 1987 read: "Jamie has had a very good first term at Terrington. He appears to be coping well with his school work and to be enjoying the new subjects he has started. Out of the form room he appears to have little trouble using his spare time profitably and I am sure will have much to contribute in years to come," (Desmond Gray).

A receipt for the Summer 1990 included the following items: Blazer, shorts, shirts, pullover, socks, rugby shirt, games socks, PE shorts, PE vests, tracksuit, sweatshirt, and dufflecoat. I soon acquired the nickname 'Castors', on account of walking round as though on wheels. This name stuck with me throughout my time at Terrington.

I have a lot of happy thoughts and memories about my time there. There were many opportunities presented to us all over the years, ranging from sport, music, drama, dance, to school trips away, including skiing in France on one occasion. There was a lot of regular competition between us and other similar schools, mainly football, rugby, athletics or cricket for the boys, and netball or rounders for the girls, and hockey and tennis for both. We would be selected for teams according to age and ability, then transported in the minibus to the venue concerned for a match; sometimes the match would be at Terrington on 'home turf' though.

Rival schools that I can remember included Grosvenor (their running star, Jamie Holmes, often won the cross-country races), Ripon Cathedral School (we once beat them 10-0 at football), Howsham Hall (they hosted an annual rugby sevens tournament; one year I was our fly-half and shouted everybody to line up. Somebody told me to shout so I promptly instructed "Shout!" to everybody. Howsham used to send their boys on a pre-breakfast wakeup run every morning); now in 2011, Howhsam is no longer a school and is for sale as a private country home for many £millions! Bramcote (strong rugby and cricket teams, including a very fast bowler), Aysgarth (William Murray, who also went to Durham after he left this school; he was a fast winger. Also, Max from Aysgarth met me on a vacation orchestral course, 'Yorchestra', (but we never kept in touch), Red House Norton (Simon Cavey was a big, fast rugby winger and he also spent five years at Durham afterwards. Now in 2010, I occasionally see his name in association with York City Rugby in local newspapers, and we are Facebook friends), Cundal Manor (Richard Wilkinson Lough was their Headboy. He came to Durham school as well for five years).

We were able to learn to swim in the fifteen metre indoor pool as well. There would be times set for swimming, and in the summer months there would be a 7am early morning swim available for those who wished, on a Wednesday. I sometimes got up especially for these sessions. Marcus Smith, David Howard, and Sarah Hartley were probably the best swimmers in school when I was there. Marcus had webbed toes and was able to swim faster as a consequence. David was the first amongst us to swim a mile, and Sarah was frequently admired in her swimming costume by the boys.

The sleeping arrangements were dormitories divided by gender and age. For boys we would start in Lawrence (bed at 7pm), then Haig (7.30pm), Annexe (7.50pm), Gort and Beatty (8pm), Jellicoe (8.15pm), Clemence (8.30pm) then Scafell (8.45 pm) for the senior boys. I can still recall Steven Lennon joking around in Jellicoe! The girls' dormitories were Claire Francis and Nightingale. Every evening the duty master and matron would ensure we were on time and brushed our teeth etc, even to the extent of a regular hygiene inspection in the bathroom. We would queue up one by one and have our feet, hands and teeth examined every night before bed. In the bathroom we shared sinks, footbaths and showers. Sometimes some of the boys would try to take a bath in the footbaths. The drying room was always very warm and occasionally boys and girls would have a secret rendezvous here.

When I started I was in Haig and once showed off to everybody by running and jumping into my bottom bunk. My head caught the bed springs and started to bleed so I had to go to 'san' for a bandage and towel to mop it up with. I got away without needing stitches, somehow. There was also a 'sick room' called

Monty, for when poorly. Here we were fed with boiled water and egg custard until better.

Maybe to compensate for being at boarding school, in the Christmas holidays, mum and dad bought me my first pet – a grey budgerigar with a blue cere ('Monty'). Monty lived for about three years before catching a fatal cold. I had a theory that it was to do with the location of the cage, which was kept in the kitchen above the deep-fat chip-pan fryer, although I was informed that the cage was moved every time the chips were made, with Monty inside. He used to sing, fly, sit on heads and shoulders, peck ears, and could say his name and also 'shut the door!'. I buried Monty amongst the fruit bushes at home.

We acquired a replacement budgerigar, a blue bird called Peter. He performed similar tricks but needed taming for some time. Peter didn't mind walking onto your finger and could say his name as well. Peter also died young at home from a cold. I was very sad about my budgerigars for quite a while.

Back at Terrington, in the senior year we got to watch the Nine o'clock News every weeknight and the school prefects could discuss the day's events afterwards. I was never elected as a prefect though. Along with many, I thought I would have made a cracking school prefect but evidently nobody else agreed. One time I was selected to be a Junior Acting Prefect but never got nominated for the full-time job.

We were taught many different subjects at school, ranging through Latin, History, Geography, Scripture, PE, Music, Art, English, Maths, French and Outdoor Pursuits. Mr John Hamer used to teach Latin and Maths. He smoked like a chimney, but had a real sense of humour and coached sport from the sidelines. He could get through to us as he was only about 5'4'' tall and didn't need to look down on us as kids. His son, Andrew, once called him 'titch' but was duly reprimanded because of this. Mr Hamer's school reports went from this 1988 Latin report: "His standard in class can be very variable; on occasions he works quite quickly and accurately but at the slightest sign of difficulty, real or imaginary, he grinds to a halt," to an improved final Latin report at Terrington in the summer of 1992: "He has worked hard this term and I was very pleased with his excellent Common Entrance result to Durham. He has always worked neatly and accurately and he fully deserved his final success. I wish him every success in the future: A+," (John Hamer).

Mr Tim Chapman taught French and coached rugby, cricket, running and football. He used to be on the pitch all the time and played for Malton and Norton Rugby Football Club, who went on to win the Championship in later years. Mr Chapman was married with young kids and used to hang out with Mr Martin Wright as well as Mr Hamer. Mr Chapman's French reports ranged from: "Jamie seems keen to learn and is interested in the subject. He has a good vocabulary," through to: "His comprehension is really improving and it is only his written work that lets him down in exams. He must make more of an effort to check every sentence for agreement."

Mr Martin Wright taught History and PE and would often come to class in a tracksuit. He used to drive a big motorbike, giving rides to his favourites, and was married to Annie the Art teacher (she took over from Fiona Wragg, who was married to John Wragg, an English teacher who used to walk around saying 'bosom, bosom'). They had a daughter called Rosie but she was at another school. Mr Hamer, Mr Chapman and Mr Wright often cracked jokes together and coached all the sport between them. Mr Wright had a proud certificate on the classroom wall for downing a yard of ale. One of his Games reports for me in 1991 read: " He can be a frustrating player as he seldom shows any signs of enjoyment. He has good qualities but these are too often hidden behind a façade of non-involvement. He should have more confidence in his abilities and not drift out of the game so much."

Another games report written by John Hamer in the Spring of 1990 read: " He has been a valuable member of the rugby team playing at full-back; his tackling has been quite sound and he has often run with speed and determination when in possession of the ball." In PE, Autumn 1989, Martin Wright wrote: "He is a spasmodic worker. He does have some talent."

The best teacher by far was Mr Tim Anderson (English). He would teach with a real flare and get us interested in learning. He also came out running with us, and helped coach rugby. Mr Anderson was in charge of Outdoor Pursuits when the time came. He had a wife and son, Edward, of whom he was very proud. He moved on to teach at a better school after several years though. Once, his wife had some serious internal bleeding and was rushed to hospital. The whole school prayed for her. She recovered. Mr Anderson once wrote of me that: "His comprehension is good, but he lacks the inclination to sparkle, hence his essays are mundane, silly or merely scruffy." Autumn 1991: " Jamie is beginning to show some sparkle in comprehension. His essays remain childish, ill thought out and hollow." Then in Spring 1992: " He is beginning to really shine at this subject. I am convinced he will do better still. (1st place with 72%)." I won the school English prize in summer 1991 – a £10 book token, and bought a fishing book from Malton.

Mr Desmond Gray was Headmaster for all my time at Terrington and his wife Gill was Headmatron. They had taken over from Mr Clementson some years previously. I always thought that as matron, she could be really demonic at times. Once I was injured on the sport's pitch and when I arrived limping at the 'san' she accused me of crying wolf. They retired to near Whitby and went on to run a Bed and Breakfast after their time at Terrington. One summer we were all invited to go on a day trip to their home near the river Esk. We were blessed with good weather and played in the garden. Mrs Gray made the boys keep short hair, so I vowed that when I grew up I would return to school one day with a head full of long hair just to make a point, but I never did. Later, at the end of January 2010, I received the sad news on Facebook that Mr Gray had had a long illness and had passed away. Even though the school was a distant memory for me I still felt emotional, as an Old Terringtonian. Some former pupils were in attendance of his funeral as well as family.

The scripture teacher was called Ted Chapman, who was also the school vicar of the local Church of England. His wife, Kath, actually died whilst I was at the school and that was also a sad time indeed.

Miss Blythe taught Geography and was quite strict at times. Once, during a morning break somebody didn't drink their milk as they should have done. She made a big thing of the spare cup, and at the end of the day kept a group of us waiting until somebody owned up. I remember Charles Saggers, Melissa Bates, Marcus Brookfield all there. Nobody knew who didn't drink it, so in the end I told her it was me, so that we could all go again. Nobody said anything afterwards, anyway. Miss Blythe once wrote of me in a school Geography report that: "His exam and early term work were still below standard but he has improved a lot recently." It was in one of Miss Blythe's early Geography lessons that I felt poorly, turned my head and vomited all over Lisa Shaw who was sitting next to me. No wonder she slammed a door in my face when I asked her out some time later.

The first Music Director during my time was Alexander Massey. Also a composer, he wrote a school musical called 'The Giant Hunder'. Charles Saggers got the lead role as the giant, although he was not very tall, so it was a joke for some time. One year, in the school play I had the role of a 'three-legged camel leader' – my only line was "a three-legged camel and a bottle of beer". Mr Massey was only nineteen years old and I think he was unpopular with other teachers for some reason. I believe he left to go to the West End to pursue a music career. Mr Massey wrote of me that: "Jamie works fast and efficiently in drama, and has produced some cleverly thought out scenes. On the piano, he now needs to look for a wider range of expression, as well as learning neater methods of practice."

The next Music Director was Geoffrey Ayling, and he taught me how to play 'Pink Panther' on piano. Autumn 1989 read: "Steady progress is being made. Particular areas for improvement just now are attention to reading skills (clefs) and to expressive elements, with a view to making his performance more interesting. His response to new ideas has been good." Ken Starks (Head of Science) taught me 'Chopsticks' one quiet afternoon. Spring 1989, Mr Starks wrote in my science report that: "Jamie is a bit of a dreamer, and there are days when his attention is obviously elsewhere. His best work is pretty good." One time he bought a black kitten from the Rymers in our village and I took it to school for him in a basket. Within two years I heard that somebody's dog had savaged the kitten and it had died. I was distraught for some time. In school concerts I played piano and viola. The maths teacher once played some ABBA tunes on the piano at my request.

Names that I can remember in my year and next, are as follows: Simon Goodrick, Marcus Smith (goalkeeper), Marc Slade, Chris Bettin, Steven and David Lennon, Tim Brampton, William Hunt, Alexander Bailey, Lisa Shaw, Kelly Gower, Carrie Magee, Clare Nelthorpe, Tom Nelthorpe, Adam Sykes, Joseph and Marcus Brookfield (their mother was a church Deacon at the time), David Downer, Zoe and Hanni Loynes (the prettiest girls in school), Michelle Wood, Bonner Earl, and Daniel Utley. Two other goalkeepers were Peter Hartley and Alan Tate-Smith (as in the soft drinks company). There were others too, some day pupils and some changing schools. Other names I recall are the Tate-Smith brothers Alan and James, David and Steven Lennon, Ben Branson, Tom Sanderson, the O'Grams David and James, James Bradley, Clare Brampton, Emma and Robert Dilger, Sean Slade, Adam Hardman, Jamie and Claire Thompson, Richard and Lorna Dale (Richard 'stole' my place as full-back on the 1st XV rugby team), Caroline and Jacqueline Redgwick, Sarah Francis, Vicky James, Joseph Sharps (whom we nicknamed 'Gold bar'), and many more worth talking about. Victoria James became the school's first Head girl the year after I left. Incidentally we once had a kiss underneath the artroom table during an evening of fun and games, and I subsequently wrote her a love letter in the school holidays but my attempt was in vain…there was to be no reply. Maybe I was a terrible kisser?

The Green Dragon

Rugby was a big thing at school. We had three main terms – Autumn (soccer), Winter (rugby), and Summer (Cricket). The three school 'houses' were Drakes, Clives, and Rhodes. I was in Drakes house. All the boys and girls were part of a 'house'. We would compete in everything over the years, ranging from chess, air-rifle shooting, tennis, rugby sevens, swimming, athletics, football and 20-20 cricket. In one match I tackled David Easterby from Rhodes house and after the match he gave me 10/10 for bravery! Drakes won the rugby sevens that year. In 1989 I was awarded four stars in a National Coca-Cola football awards scheme. Everyone in school was awarded something, with five stars being the highest available.

In my final year there was to be a school football tour across to Merseyside. Some allegation had been made against me that I had said 'girls are rubbish' or something. Martin Wright dropped me from the squad because of the allegation. I never went on that tour, but the Terrington team got hammered every single match they played. They told me they got to watch a premiership match involving Everton as well when they got back. I didn't feel too upset about that incident.

My last sports day made up for that, anyway. I entered the 800 metres, 400 metres, triple jump, javelin, and house relay. Out of those five I ended up with four gold medals and one silver – with Drakes just seconded in the relay. Also I broke the 1991 school triple jump record. I wonder if this still stands? Mum and Dad had witnessed the occasion and my friend Marc Slade had also won all his events, too; 100 metres, 200 metres, high jump, shot put, and relay. His dad was a PE instructor in the army, which Marc went on to join in later years, also playing as much football as possible along the way. In the summer holidays I went to visit Marc near Weymouth. His dad, Jim Slade, picked me up from Honiton station on a big sports motorbike and drove me back to their home at the barracks. Marc also accompanied me on holiday to my Uncle Rob's in Cornwall one time in the summer. Another year Daniel Utley came along to Cornwall. Uncle Rob and Aunty Wendy have lived in numerous properties, but at this time they lived in a beautiful big house called Trethowa with an outdoor swimming pool and boat and huge garden, etc. We were privileged indeed to visit. Matthew and Helen were their offspring – two of my six cousins.

Every year towards the end of the summer term there were school photographs taken for all sorts of groups and teams representing the entire year. I did have lots but in later years my school pictures were misplaced or damaged, and very few remain now. Steve Lennon generously posted some Terrington photos on my Facebook page in 2009 which brought back some memories. School reports were issued at the end of every term. They also became misplaced over the years.

I once won the school clay pigeon shooting competition. Nick Robshaw came a close second. Technically I won on theory points and he won on practical, but the combined components of shooting and theory test put me ahead! In my final year I got to the tennis singles final but Christopher Howard beat me. I won the doubles with Marcus Smith, though. In table tennis, Andrew Room won the main tournament (he was nicknamed 'Digger' for some reason). I won the runners-up tournament.

For a year, when I was 12, I 'went out' with Carrie Magee. We both had a crush on each other. Her dad Ralph, once took a small group of us to the Houses of Parliament in London to meet John Greenway – Conservative MP. I was there along with Claire Nelthorpe, Bonner Earle and Carrie. I was the only 'non-prefect' of the four of us. Ralph's secretary, Elaine also attended, and was involved in the divorce of Carrie's parents. Elaine eloped with Ralph to detrimental effect. He also owned a hot air balloon and a biscuit factory. Carrie had two younger brothers, Chris and Matthew. She was swimming one afternoon and I was outside messing round. I knocked on the pool window to speak to her, then she decided to get changed and meet me. We sneaked into the music room locker room and kissed for a while. It was my first proper kiss and I remember being really grossed out by it at the time. They lived in a big house in West Lilling near Sheriff Hutton and owned a swimming pool as well.

The Green Dragon

There were always boys and girls chasing each other, and various crushes materialising. We would sometimes arrange to meet on the school sports field by the 'love machine'. Actually it was a grass-roller machine, but we liked to call it that. I think it was William Pexton who came up with that name. Other times, people met in the Walled garden where some were granted a personal allotment for vegetables or plants. I used to grow carrots, radishes, lettuce, and pumpkins. Plus I kept a compost heap for peeing onto.

The senior common room for the pupils was the old English Room. We each had a locker in there and boys and girls could mix in their spare time. I kept my fishing tackle up there and there were always Nintendo Gameboys being passed around to play on and various cd's being played on the stereo, ranging from Guns 'n' Roses, Madness, Madonna, Dire Straits, Whitesnake, Queen, U2, INXS, and Elton John, to Richard Marx, as well as other games invented ranging from how long you could make a Cadbury's cream egg last, to more risky spin the bottle truth or dare.

While I was at Terrington, Mum and Dad bought me a computer – my very own Commodore 64, complete with Kickstart, Pit Stop 2, the Last Ninja 2, Paradroid, Run the Gauntlet, the Summer Games, and many other games, too. My brother Jonny tried his hand at computer programming on the Commodore 64. We would often compete at different games over the years. At school all the other kids wanted a turn as well.

Some of us went on fishing trips to the local Wiganthorpe lake in summer months. This would involve carting our tackle across several fields and walking for twenty minutes cross-country to get there. I only ever caught small roach and tench. I nearly caught a pike once but it got away. David Easterby held the school record for catching the biggest pike from Wiganthorpe lake. He carried it back to school and the kitchen staff served it up for his table that evening.

Other local lakes were at Castle Howard and Birkdale farm. I once fished at Castle Howard and caught nothing. Ian Botham presented the winner with a prize and the whole event raised funds for 'Heartclick' charity. Mum had come to watch all day which helped, but I had to borrow a keep-net from a fellow-angler as I only had a landing net. Tim Brampton and myself often went to Birkdale lake in the school holidays and went night-fishing for carp, tench or other freshwater species. The record held was by Tim who caught a 4lb Mirror Carp late one night. We used to set up a tent, and wear my father's ex-RAF bomber crew flying suits to keep warm in the early hours. We must have looked a right pair if anyone saw us in the dark! One morning we were packing up and Tim accidentally stuck the boilie-baiter hook into his finger. My brother Jonny arrived in the car and drove him to the local Dr Bradley's surgery to have it removed surgically. Ouch!!!!

I once had an outrageous crush on a Maths teacher. She was blonde and gorgeous, and good at maths. She actually left the school before long so I never got a look in. Maybe I was too young after all, though. An assistant Corrine Johnson gave me a birthday kiss, but that was because I insisted and some of my friends also insisted on my behalf. That set me up for months!

In the summer term, on a Sunday, there were sometimes 'walking picnics' taking place. We were driven maybe five miles into the countryside and dropped in groups of 4-6 people, then left to make our own way back to school with a picnic for sustenance. So long as we signed back in again that was all that mattered. Ken Starks was the science teacher in charge of our walking picnics. We used to nickname him 'carrots' for some reason.

For the boarders, Saturday night was movie night. We would sit in the living room in our pyjamas and watch the movie of choice. I can remember watching 'Mad Max in Thunderdome' starring Mel Gibson and Tina Turner. I was with Carrie at the time.

The Green Dragon

Moneywise, I didn't receive much at all. £5 a term, to put a figure on it. On a Wednesday morning break we were allowed 50 pence to go to the village shop for sweets, and on a Sunday 20 pence for sweets and 20 pence to give to the local church. So, on a budget of less than £1 a week I spent my entire five years like this. Letters from home went on display in the corridor every morning. I used to look forwards to receiving post. On a Sunday we had to write two letters to relatives every week. I used to write home and to my grandparents.

Mum and Dad were both music teachers at Terrington and would come to the school one or two days every week to teach. Dad taught woodwind and brass instruments ranging from trumpet to oboe, or clarinet and saxophone, and mum taught piano, and flute. I began taking lessons in piano with Mr Alexander Massey at first until he left as music director after a few years. Then Mr Geoffrey Ayling took over and he taught me piano, although I didn't much enjoy it at the time. Mrs Jill Bowman taught me violin but I decided I preferred viola as the tone was deeper and more satisfying to listen to. Mum drove me to Jill's house (then in Gilling East) every week for a lesson. I also got to play with her son and daughter at these times, too: Jonan and Ruth. They were at school in York, so we were at different schools, but our paths crossed again in later years.

Some pupils were selected for the school choir. We would rehearse during the week, and then on Sunday we had to wear a red and white cassock to the local church service and sing from the stalls in front of everybody in the congregation. We were always given a liquorice sweet to warm up our vocal chords by the vicar before the service. We would take it in turns to ring the bells for the service, but usually would swing from the ropes.

Meals at Terrington were threefold. Breakfast was the first event of every day after getting up and dressed. Lunch was after morning lessons, with a mid-morning snack offered during the break period. Then after lunch we had games outdoors for a while, then changed in the changing rooms for lessons once again. These changing rooms were the scene of many a fun n games session during our spare time, ranging from 'escape from Colditz', to general sports shenanigans. Then on an evening we would have tea in the dining room. Each boarder was granted a 'goody tin' at the beginning of term, for teatime. Two plates were placed on each table from that table's goody tins and we would share cake or biscuits like this.

The annual Christmas dinner was a grand occasion in December. The whole school turned up and speeches were made by the masters, and jokes cracked. Then we would go to the hall for entertainment, either magic or music, for an hour. This was really a great thing to look forward to. Mr Anderson used to try and teach us grammar in an elaborate and gesticulative manner at this event.

School fights did happen but I can remember only a few towards the end of my time there. Jonathan Price once accosted me for some reason, and I gave him a hard knee in the groin as a gut reaction. He didn't do it again. Another time, I was in the changing rooms and admiring my new penknife. Matthew Sampson was disparaging about it, and I again reacted instinctively, and punched him in the head. He then reacted and picked up a cricket stump and brandished it fiercely. He must have drunk a Castlemaine XXXX, or a Fosters that day! He was Australian. Mr Hamer appeared from somewhere and calmed the situation down. Nobody ever told me off for that even though Matthew was bruised for a week.

Once, at Tim Brampton's house in Kirby, some village kids suddenly appeared in the garden one day and determined to set upon us. They said they only wanted to fight me really but I was not willing to fight them. Tim got drawn into a fist fight with two other kids and then they left as suddenly as they had appeared. Tim and I were more interested in cycling and fishing than fighting. One morning at 5am we got up and took his parents' tandem for a spin round the quiet streets of Kirkbymoorside. Other times we would challenge each other to see how long we could stay awake on a nighttime whilst watching telly or listening to records. Both our families took it in turns to book a villa at Sherwood Forest Center Parc in the holidays. We swam in the rapids, played snooker and badminton, fished for trout, went out on a pedalo, biked everywhere. We met Eleanor in the swimming pool and exchanged villa numbers. Eleanor was older than Tim and I and lived in Harrogate. We tried to phone up after the holiday, but it soon fell through after some stern words from her father. Tim and I went fishing a lot. That was our main activity other than cycling. Other times we cycled to Nunnington Hall, aged 10-12, and enjoyed cream teas. We really lived it up at that age, man! Whilst boarding at school, one windy, rainy night in Jellico, Tim made everyone laugh when he stuck his head out of the window and started shouting to some village kid: "We worship the wind and the rain, Hare Krishna, Hare, Hare!" Tim was probably my best friend from Terrington. After we left school we were briefly reunited at Durham school for a while, but that didn't work out because he left. Then round about 2010 we reunited on Facebook, amongst many other of our friends. It wasn't until August 2010 that we actually met up for a drink at the Blues Club in Scarborough. There we enjoyed the music, and another Kirkbymoorside friend – Charles Dale, mentioned in chapter three, came out too, along with Scarborough Dave. They were interested in my first book – Plan 103f. The three of us went to London's West End to watch the musical 'Blood Brothers' in October 2010. We went to the Phoenix Theatre with Alex Boorman, too, who was to be my Best Man the next month (November 2010).

Other school fights I remember were Marcus Smith and Marc Slade scrapping on the playing fields in front of everybody for some reason, and another time Chris Bettin and Marc Slade boxing in our common room. I was pretending to be some kind of coach to Chris Bettin.

Another daft thing that happened was with Adam Sykes. One night in Haig dormitory the other boys dared us to bounce our bum cheeks together. Rumours set off after that for a while. Seemed funny at the time.

I used to hang out with Tim, Daniel Utley, Marcus Smith, and Marc Slade. Tim and Marc tried to smoke rolled up teabags at one point, but I wasn't bothered by this. I used to fancy Michelle Wood like crazy. Tim's sister Clare once helped me write a letter to her and send a miniature sparkler 'to celebrate our love'. I never got a reply for some reason. Apparently the sparkler had crumbled into pieces by the time she got the letter in the post.

In the summer holidays, mum used to take us to Cornwall to stay with my uncle for a fortnight. He lived in various locations over the years, throughout Cornwall and Devon, along with Aunty Wendy and my cousins Matthew and Helen. The first time I can recall Cornwall was when they lived on a farm near Penzance, called 'Sunnymeade'. I can remember the big John Deere tractor, the stacks of hay bales in the barn, the livestock in the fields, shooting Matt's Gat airgun in the orchard, mackerel fishing around St Michael's Mount in Uncle Rob's boat with mackerel feathers, listening to a record called 'Hurdy gurdy mushroom man' by Neale, and a BMX track in a small village called 'Mousehole' where I fell backwards off the starting blocks and split my head open. It bled for a while but soon healed. Matthew was into surfing from an early age and in later years went on to manage his own Cornish beach near Newquay and was frequently found cheffing in various hotels, restaurants and pubs around the world. Helen was older and I remember she never liked me too much, and once I told her off for smoking but got told where to go (at Sunnymeade). I acquired a special t-shirt from St Ives which stated that "I don't look for trouble, trouble finds me!" This has kind of remained the case throughout my life!

The drive from Yorkshire to Penzance took about ten hours, so Mum would often stop at Grandma and Grandad's home in Bromsgrove for the night (8 Leadbetter Drive), and visit Uncle Andy, Aunty Ricky, Christiana and Antonia en route, too, in their home near Redditch. They owned a swimming pool and my Uncle Andy managed a big car showroom garage for about twenty years or so. Aunty Ricky had horse-riding stables close

The Green Dragon

by as well. Both Christiana and Antonia went on to strive for and experience great success in life in various fields including tennis, athletics/cross country running, medicine and cycling. They both worked very hard, played hard, and thoroughly deserved everything in life. I wish that we could have a family reunion one day in decent circumstances. Once when we visited on these trips, I had a skin disease called 'impetigo' and wasn't allowed in the house so I was left on the garden swings for an hour on my own while everyone else talked inside.

Uncle Rob then moved to another huge house near Truro called 'Trethowa', with Aunty Wendy, Matthew, Helen, big garden, boat named 'Redwing', swimming pool and an English sheepdog called Ben. Matthew owned his first car by then, a VW Beetle. Helen worked in hotels as a receptionist. Alternate years I invited a school friend to come with us - Daniel Utley and Marc Slade. We used to go hunting rabbits with our air rifles, once coming home with half a dozen on a stick. We played tennis in Truro, and went out in Rob's boat to catch mackerel at sea, or trout in a lake. Other times we went to the beach to go body-boarding and chill out in the sun and get a tan. Marc and I used to go on training runs for between 3-5 miles sometimes, on a morning. I discovered I could do press-ups at that age. On an evening we used to sit in the living room and Aunty Wendy would tell us funny stories. Matthew always had time for us when we went there, cavorting and carrying on, etc. I can remember the buskers in Truro and the cathedral. Mum would always shop at Tesco. We (the boys) stayed in the garden caravan whilst Mum had a luxury ensuite room inside. There I had acquired another special t-shirt with an image of Sylvester the cat and the words "Rebel without claws". We were very lucky to be there!

Marc's dad – a PE instructor in the army – once picked me up at Honiton station on a big Suzuki road bike, and I then spent a week at the barracks at their place. We rode bikes and played indoor football but I badly strained a leg muscle and had to get an ice pack. Marc's younger brother Sean was also into sport. He once had ear gromits, though, and had to have an operation. He also had a nasty bike accident and broke his arm.

Back up north again, my first trips to France were from Terrington. One summer the Kershaws and the Bowmans went on a joint trip to spend a week on a French barge. We met at the canal in Paris, on the river Seine, and David (Mr Bowman) was the ship's captain for the week. Every morning we would have baguettes from the local boulangerie and every evening we would tie up ship and bunk down. I remember the strawberry cheese we discovered in a restaurant along the riverside one evening. We had bikes hired out, too, for some parts. Chris (my eldest brother) was in charge of roping the boat at locks, and sometimes we spent hours waiting for the barge to pass through the locks. My 'holiday handiwork' was to write about this holiday experience and share the tale with others back home.

The other trip to France was a school skiing trip. The bus left Terrington one evening and we travelled overnight to Grenoble. I think we must have caught an aeroplane because I remember a group of us meeting the pilot and receiving a badge. We stayed in a chalet and I shared with my mum. Dr Bradley (GP) had organised the whole trip; her son, James, was a little younger than myself. They also had their own private tennis court back home. I remember skiing with Oliver Mackereth and Charles Lamb, who wore a lucky rabbit's foot on his crash helmet. Charles Lamb was one of the more intelligent pupils at school, always showing off his vocabulary, along with Joseph Sharps, who enjoyed eating white chocolate 'gold bars'.

Dr Bradley had the job of vaccinating the entire school with a flu jab in winter months, then handing out free lollies afterwards. At an early age I suffered from eczema, asthma, impetigo, nits, warts, athlete's foot and conjunctivitis. Trips to the school san kept us healthy. I remember the 'new skin' lotion for my athlete's foot really stinging when applied. It worked, though.

Another foreign experience came in 1991, when I went to Bergen, Norway, with my dad for an annual Esperanto congress. My dad spoke and taught the language enthusiastically and thought it would be an idea to take me along to an international congress. We caught the plane from Newcastle to Bergen, then spent a week in student lodgings, but all I remember now is lots of people from all round the world gathering in the 'Grieg-Hallen' and attending events/concerts/dinners/excursions/ talks. I was trying to meet other similar-aged kids as well. It seemed exciting to go abroad for a week and it was then that I learnt that the composer, Grieg, was Norwegian, and I sampled Scandinavian ale which dad said was very expensive. The only words I actually said in Esperanto to the adults who spoke to me were "Iom ete" (meaning "a little"), usually in reply to the question "Ĉu vi parolas Esperanton?" We went on boats, ferries around some fjords, and then a mountain bus trip which was hair-raising at times owing to narrow passes and traffic trying to get past. Dad once left a complaint note on the residence door about the students' music being too loud on a night. The note didn't last very long and the music kept on playing. Our flight back to Newcastle, UK, was straightforward, with eldest brother Chris meeting us in a car with then girlfriend Nicola.

I could be really moody at times. One time in a five-a-side football tournament I was given the 'yellow card' by David O'Gram. I sulked, then got sent off completely. It was all too much for me. Other times in the school hall we had games of five-a-side football and 'pirates and coastguards'. The 16-year-old kitchen assistant enjoyed playing football with us but I don't remember his name now.

The school had a brand new teaching block built whilst I was there - five new classrooms and a store room facing the front garden. We had previously used this area for practising our fishing casting on the lawn.

In the summer months we were allowed to bring our bikes to school and keep them underneath the changing rooms in the basement. We would ride around the playing fields and later on even rode ten miles home with friends. And after the weekend we would cycle back to school again on a Sunday evening in time for school the next day. Marc Slade, Tim Brampton, and I made this journey several times. Tim's family lived in Kirbymoorside.

Daniel Utley had an elder brother Jacob, and a younger sister Harriet. They lived in Pontefract, West Yorkshire. Sometimes in the holidays we stayed over at each other's houses, involving our parents driving a long way! Air rifle shooting, fishing and some basic hunting skills were of interest. Daniel had an entire taxidermy collection of stuffed birds and animals in his bedroom. Sometimes we stayed in their caravan. They lived near Pontefract race course, so we ran round it on occasion, and near a Haribo sweet factory, where I tried 'Pontefract cakes'.

An annual summertime event was the Under-eleven's cricket match versus our mothers. Mum never forgave me for bowling her out first ball at that match. I also bowled out Mrs Woolsey but the umpire (Mr Hamer) called 'no ball!' so that her son – Chris – could bowl instead. I never got too much into cricket, anyway.

Three big events that everybody in school looked forward to were the Wye river canoe trip, the Seniors' Lake District trip, and the leavers' barbecue. Fifth form went to the river Wye for a week in the holidays. We canoed fifty miles from Hereford to Monmouth over three to five days. Each day Mr and Mrs Gray packed the entire camp up into the minibuses and drove to the next campsite further downriver. We would have competitions en route and raft up, capsize, walk over each others' canoes etc. Jacob Utley (Daniel's older brother) came back to canoe with our year.

Symonds Yat was a stretch of white water rapids which we feared greatly but once we got there we had to go individually and meet at the bottom of the stretch. Some people capsized and others didn't. We were wearing lifejackets and helmets so nobody could actually drown. I managed to keep my balance here and got through the rapids in one piece, thankfully. This was a highlight of the Wye trip. We were blessed with group leaders from the army, and every evening we sat round the tent and ate, drank and shared stories and jokes. I shared a tent with Simon Goodrick because we both had asthma so needed non-feather sleeping bags.

The Lake District trip was in the final year. We were driven to the campsite near lake Buttermere. The farmhouse there served as our headquarters. For one week we were divided into groups and spent our daytimes sailing, rock-climbing and hiking/walking. Kiffy James came back as a previous leaver to help with these expeditions. He was Vicky James' elder brother. We moved campsites as we walked, literally carrying camp with us. One night I had bad asthma and Lisa Shaw had me take an inhaler, so I could breathe properly again after a few minutes. This trip was exhausting and drenching as the weather fluctuated between warm and dry, and cold and wet. This was another highlight of my time at Terrington Hall!

Two later Headmaster's reports read (Spring 1990) that: "Jamie makes steady progress but somehow I have the feeling that there is more to him than we have seen so far. There have been glimpses of a real determination once or twice on the games field which I hope we will soon see in both his work and music." And the final 1992 report at Terrington read: "Jamie is to be congratulated on an excellent result in Common Entrance and it underlines the ability we always knew he possessed. He should be able to get into a good set at Durham and I hope that will encourage him to work hard and achieve the success I know him to be capable of. I wish Jamie every success for the future and will follow his progress at Durham with interest," (Desmond Gray).

The leavers' barbecue was the last chance our year would ever have to be together, having spent the best part of five years growing up and developing together. The leavers of the year could cook the barbecue and even drink an alcoholic beverage if they so desired. Mr Gray handed us each a leaver's tie to keep. Afterwards we threw each other into the swimming pool fully-clothed and smashed some windows in what was the disused chapel on the playing fields. This was our goodbye to our time at Terrington, and there were tears as well as smiles and laughter.

After I had left, the only time I ever visited the school again was as an eighteen year old. I had finished at Durham and was about to travel around Europe, inter-railing, for the summer of 1997. On my way to York station I called in and briefly spoke to Mr Hamer, Mr and Mrs Gray, and Mr Chapman in the dinner hall at lunchtime. They had all remembered me even though totally surprised by my being there again after all those years. I hope that the kids didn't mind too much! This was the last time I ever spoke to Mr Gray.

The summer holiday interim between Terrington and Durham school was spent on a youth orchestral course called 'Yorchestra', in York, the city of my birth. There my parents paid for me playing viola for a week, and met the other kids. I was very shy most of the time, and not a very good viola player. I did get a prize for 'best player', though it was really for hitting a home run in a game of softball. I can remember Jonan Bowman (cello), Juliet Bedford (clarinet), Hannah Teale (cello), Mark G Caroll (cello), Annabel Trapp (violin), et al. One lunchbreak I was sitting outside with all the other kids and a wasp chose to fly down the back of my shirt and sting me. I panicked and cried. One of the coaches calmed me down again. Very professional!

Although born in York, I never went to school, lived, or worked in York. The viola coach, Pauline, used to laugh gleefully whenever she made me smile. In later years (aged 17) I dated Hannah for aout a year, although at college in different cities. Then, in 2010, I remet Mark G Caroll on the internet social network Facebook. Much water had passed under the bridge since last we spoke! Juliet talked to me as though I was normal which was nice; She went to Bootham school, York, then onto Worcester College, at Oxford University. We remained friends although at different schools until the age of eighteen. We dated in York once, maybe twice, but life moved us apart.

Chapter Two
Durham School

I spent five years of my life at Durham School, aged 13-18. My first year was known as 'Shell': September 1992-July 1993, then 'Lower V': September 1993-July 1994, then GCSE year in 'Upper V': September 1994- July 1995. Then, aged sixteen, I could legally have left school, gone to York or stayed to do A-levels. I stayed. 'Lower VI': September 1995-July 1996 was followed by 'Upper VI': September 1996-July 1997 when I took four A levels. In terms of passing 10 GCSE's and 4 A-levels, my time at Durham was a success. Otherwise, please read on for the full story.

There were three main reasons why I ended up at Durham School. 1) Offered a Teacher-assisted place for five years (parents were school teachers so qualified for the award). 2) Offered a Music Exhibition from Terrington to Durham (piano, viola, singing). 3) Mum had connections with the Bloore family, whose boys (Andrew and Robert – Poole House) had both succeeded from Terrington to Durham before I got there. I didn't particularly want to go to a town school, but we could afford it and it was an opportunity for a good schooling. Two other boys from Terrington to Durham, years before me, were Andrew Reader (School House), and Robert Penty (Poole House). Andrew was a senior 1st XV rugby player when I arrived. He used to give me Chinese burns on my arms for fun.

The first night in the dormitory, I was pretty nervous. The other boarders in my year, age 13, were Alistair Lowe, Luke Hunter-Pattinson, Ed Halford, Reetesh Saraf, Daniel Tang, and others, too, whom I can't recall now. Richard Gilbert came to Durham School as a boarder in my third year at the school. Day pupils in my year were Rupert Ellis (sharing the exact same birthday as myself), Elliott Brown, Simon Birtwhistle, Richard Gatland, Steven Riley, David Lascelles, David Curry, et al. Some of these I am now in touch with on Facebook (2011), also Simon Reay of Langley House. Alistair ended up as Head of House in our final year there, and Elliott was Deputy Headboy. I had some 'teething' squabbles with Reetesh and Daniel in my first year, resulting in a smashed clock and a threat of being covered in toothpaste. However, the school was highly multi-cultural and diverse in its approach to different subjects.

School House, aka 'Bungites', had won most inter-school sports tournaments for over 10 years since Mr Hugh Dias had been Housemaster. I was initially shown around Caffinites house, but decided I would prefer School House for some reason. There were four main boys' houses: School, Caffinites, Poole, and Langley (day pupils only), a junior house, Ferens, and a girls' house, Pimlico. I was shown Caffinites because of their musical emphasis, as opposed to School's sports emphasis. In the tournaments, School wore Blue, Caffinites Red, Poole Black, and Langley Green.

The first two years there we had a Prep hall for both years to share during daytime and evening. There were beatings and punishments issued every day for various targets from the senior boys, along with homework. Also on the good side - table tennis, daily newspapers, fruit and milk were delivered. 'Shell' members were expected to be on house delivery duty at 7 am. One boarder would have to get up early to deliver the milk to each study room, and another would have to ring the handbell at 7.30am to wake everyone up. In the year above I can remember Phil Hunter, Giles Chadwick, Michael Ainsley, Adam Brown, and Gareth Blackbird (whose elder brother Nigel frequently picked on him). Gareth had become Head of school 1995-96 by the time he left.

School meals occurred three times a day in the 'Big School' hall. Breakfast for boarders was typically between 7.45am-8.15am – usually a decent selection of food combinations - then roll call assemblies back in the individual houses at 8.20am, then daily chapel 8.35-8.55am. Each house had approximately 100 pupils. Lunch was 1pm-1.30pm, and dinner 7pm-7.30pm which occurred between compulsory prep sessions (6-7pm, then 7.45-9pm).

Bed times started with Shell 10.15pm, Lower V 10.30pm, Upper V 10.45pm, Lower VI 11pm, and Upper VI not specified. We had to be in bed for lights-out, which either a duty Master or senior monitor performed. At that time our School Music Director, Jonny Newell, was also House Tutor to School House (Bungites), so he often went around on lights-out duty. Today, he is listed amongst my Facebook friends. Matron looked after all of us, but some ruder boys used to tease her on account of her having a big bottom. She was very helpful about my asthma. Mr Hugh Dias - Housemaster – was always informed if anything happened around the house. Rugby and cricket were big things at Durham school. I wanted to be full back or winger, but got placed as Flanker on the B team. I broke my left thumb in a school match in a tackle. The nearest competing schools were Barnard Castle, and Newcastle schools.

I used to exercise before bed, doing pressups and situps. At most, 3 lots of 20 press ups in different postures, so 60 on a night, plus the same number of sit-ups when really fit. Mr Mick Hirsch – the school fitness expert from Australia - had recommended extra exercise as he was a pushy coach and had played cricket for Australia. Mr Lurch (Australian) was a temporary house assistant. Mr Andrew Zafer (Australian) took over in my latter years there and married the art teacher Miss Kim Watton. I used to have a crush on her in art lessons. She picked up on it and called me a slimeball. People used to exaggerate about the size of my nose, and I acquired the nickname 'Blair' after a character in the failed Spanish soap opera 'Eldorado' – nothing to do with Tony Blair, though it would have been good!

At Durham, my first three years were all boys, until Sixth form, when girls were equally admitted to the school. They did this so we could focus on our work and sports interests etc. I didn't want to let people down, and soon discovered that I was good at distance running after an initial training run as a group for 3.5 miles. In my Shell year I came 2nd in the Junior Kingston to Nigel Dolman, and 4th in the Junior Swainston 4½ miles. I was awarded half house colours for this – a blue/black striped tie. On my first Sports day I entered 800m, 1500m, and triple jump, and won all 3 events. Gareth Blackbird was encouraging from then on, along with other more senior boys.

Also in Sport our first rugby coach was Mr David Crook (Head of Modern languages), swimming - Mr Mick Hirsch (Cricket coach), athletics - Mr Mark Bushnell (Economics) and middle distance coach, (also Mr Paul O'Connor (History) & Mr Dougall). Nick Willings was Head of Sport and some nicknamed him 'Mouldy' for some reason. Dominic Parker and Alistair Rose were the fastest two senior racers, and I used to look up to them when they ran.

The Music Director, Mr Jonathan Newell, had granted me a Music Exhibition to the school (viola, piano, singing), and gave me a choir audition and an orchestral place, and taught classroom music ranging from group rapping to individual music projects (I opted for stringed instruments). Marc Blenkiron was our year's piano expert. Robert Ainsley was in the year above and presided on piano, organ, and violin, as well as helping conduct the school orchestra. Robert went on to Cambridge University after Durham. Mr Newell smoked a lot, drank and drove fast cars saying: "If you've gotta go, go in style". I struggled to learn piano. My teacher Miss Jackie Thomason laughed at me as I got the wrong notes. One evening whilst practising in the music school, Stuart Connelly observed me and said to keep it up. He was the best at javelin in the school, and a sprinter, met his girlfriend in sixth form and joined the RAF.

Other subjects in my Shell year included 'Art' with Mr Malia (also a rugby coach and head of expeditions), and Miss Kim Watton (wanted me to do GCSE art but I chose music instead). English was with Mr Hugh Dias, Geography with Mr Renshaw, to whom I once piped up, "Nice day, ain't it sir!" He corrected my bad English at the time and every one laughed in class. French with Mr David Crook (went on to become Head of Languages, aka 'the Boss'), CDT with the stern Mr Fred Cook (also cross-country coach), Latin with Mr Bucholdt (I cried in class once owing to being bullied as a boarder, and he got people

The Green Dragon

told off), Maths with Miss Jenny Growcott (joined the RAF in later years), Scripture with Mrs Proud (son Steven a cellist, and daughter Claire an Organ scholar), and History with Mr Hind (bell ringer/campanologist). My first year reports were a bit behind, mostly with Cs and Ds, but my athletics made up for that in the eyes of others. Nick Vise taught French and Spanish and became a father during my time at Durham; he was also the School House assistant after Jonny Newell had moved on. Nick Hill was Music Assistant-Director, and Caffinites Duty Master. Mr Hill left Durham school to be Music Director elsewhere.

An early 'Shell' report for French read: "He has worked steadily throughout the term and his examination result of 73% is to his credit. Of late he has put a little more energy into class participation and I would like to see this continue. A promising linguist!" And in Lower V my French teacher wrote: "He is doing well but he should aim to be the best if he can. I know that he will rise to the challenge," (D M Crook).

We were drafted into the school CCF where we did marching, shooting, etc, and had to choose between the RAF, Navy, or Army. I opted for the RAF as my father had been in the RAF as a Radar Fitter. I didn't much like CCF but got to fly in gliders twice, and I was amongst the last people ever to fly in a Chipmunk aircraft. Henry Gatland was always very encouraging about the CCF, even though he laughed at my daft marching. I never wanted to join the army, navy or air force after school, though. My cousin Jonty had been in the RAF as an administrator for a short time.

In my Lower V year I improved positions, coming 2nd to William Bishop in the Swainston 4½ miler, and winning the 800m and 1500m at sports day. There was a new lineup in the rollcall assembly room; we had moved up a year and got moved into a new dormitory, too. Once in the prep hall, Henry Collins pinched my diary so I rugby tackled him to get it back. He was an ice hockey player and often went to practise at the city ice arena.

Our dorm monitors included John Windows (brother of Richard, and 1st XV rugby scrum half. He once peed in a dorm bin after a late night out), Christopher Scott (Head of School House), John North (seeing Nicola Seaman), Martin Shaw (1st XV rugby), and David Errington (wore leather trousers for comic relief).

During the winter holidays that year, my mum took me and my brother Jonny on a skiing holiday to Austria's 'Pitztal' glacier. We caught an overnight coach from Harrogate dry ski centre and met up with Tom Williams, Jenny Elm and someone called Sarah. During the week's vacation we hung out and skied together. Tom dared me to do a black level run and I shat myself but managed to ski down without falling over, on the hard, fast, icy slopes. Tom got together with Sarah during the week.

Fighting amongst boys in the prep hall saw Ed Halford and Dan Morgan fighting hard one time. Ed and I used to play 'dead arms' in the prep hall, causing much amusement. We took it in turns to punch each other's arms to see who could take the most, and ended up badly bruised. Once I raided a dormitory after lights out and blasted everyone hard with a pillow. In my sixth form years, Jonathan Lascelles and Will Halford once fought outside a pub in the city. People used to nickname Will 'Merrick' and he didn't take it lightly. One winter term, on a snow-covered rugby pitch one evening, Richard Windle started a snowball fight. I joined in and somehow got in a tussle with one of the rugby players called Robbie. He flattened me in the snow and I tried to shrug it off by saying 'Not worth it.' That upset him worse.

Graham Unwin used to start kicking and swearing in the TV lounge. We had a snooker table, and a piano beneath the TV lounge/library. 'Bungites' was the nickname for School house. I once got locked in a corridor locker and was laughed at when I got out. Murray Wickman once played a knife game with my hand where I had to hold it still as he banged the knife between my fingers one by one. I felt a bit nervous about that one.

The Green Dragon

Other boys in that year and the younger year with whom I got on were: Mark Nixon (Poole), Alex Lowrie (Langley), Ian and Jamie Laidler (Caffinites – Ian had the nickname of 'Leggy'), Michael Ellis (Poole), Mark Simms (left after GCSEs), Paul Watson (Caffinites), Andrew Bayles (Poole, Head of school in my year), Philip Osbourne (Poole), Simon Reay (Langley), Daniel Newton, Simon Shaw (Caffinites and witness to my proudest rugby tackle in a school match), Chris Cartner (School), Gareth Jones (Poole), Matthew Courtney (Poole), Michael Goldsmith (Caffinites), Steven Coleman (Caffinites), Christopher Hilton (Langley), Paul de Cates (Caffinites with talents in Taekwondo, journalism, guitar and saxophone; he got into Oxford Uni), some of whom I am connected to today (2011) by the internet social network Facebook. Michael Liddle was a year above me, but always excelled in the Music Department.

That summer holiday I was invited to Ibiza for two weeks with Andy Millson (Caffinites) and family, when I was 15. He intended to invite Luke Hunter Patterson, but Luke had turned the invitation down for some reason. Whilst on the Balearic Island we met Kelly from Bristol. Andy's younger brother Martin, dad Steve, and mum, put me up in their hotel room for the holiday. We would split up in the day time and meet on an evening for a family meal out, etc. I went off with Andy, swimming in the sea, exploring and nosing round the markets. One time we all went on a bus ride to the hippy market and came back with some interesting items. One night Andy's parents decided to take us all to the famous casino for a night of entertainment and champagne. They won two big bottles on a game of roulette and we all got plastered. His mum was chosen from the entire audience to go on stage as the hypnotist's subject. She acted as though her chair was electrifying her bottom and couldn't stop laughing. Some nights later I tried swordfish for the first and only time in my life. It tasted a bit like chicken. We went on walks and one time walked up through the old town to the scenic area at the top of the hill.

We often went out to the Bull Bar where there was sangria on tap, a mechanical bull and a bungee run. One night on the walk back to the hotel we were attacked on the beach by a group of older Spanish blokes. They were drunk and saw we were having a good time. Andy got hurt that night. Somebody witnessed the scene from the look-off wall and started shouting for them to stop. We were shaken up for several days, and that ruined the holiday for me. But other good events there were champagne-diving from a touring boat where 10 bottles of champagne were thrown over the side and we had to dive in to get them to keep. I retrieved a bottle, and Andy retrieved three! There was also plenty of swimming, sunbathing, eating out and water-skiing for Andy and his dad doing a double act. Before he left Durham school at 16, Andy and I used to train together, running and racing to get fit.

At school, a House tutor's report by Mr Newell read: "He has opened up this term and had become quite a character in his year group, displaying zany wit on occasion!"

Back at Durham for the Upper V year, I took GCSEs in English Language and Literature, Maths, Music, French, Biology, Physics, Chemistry, PE, and ended up passing all at grades A-C. I had County trials for Durham cross country and came 4th in the Durham city schools' race. At Gateshead International stadium I got my best-ever 800metres time– 2mins 12 secs during a school meet. I never would make the Olympic Games after all! The Dunelmian run at school was for the seniors aged 16yrs+. In my first 10-miler I came 2nd to William Bishop again, about a 54 minute run. One of his trainers came off half way but he never stopped, and was on crutches for weeks afterwards. In the Intermediate Kingston I won, I came 1st! Unfortunately I had no notion of real world athletics so I was very much living within the school gates. If I could have understood about World Champions, Olympic and Commonwealth Games my life would have had a different focus and been more athletic-based. The school games report for me that term read: "He has run exceedingly well this season, and has shown with running for Durham Area that he has the potential to get onto the County team next year. Within the school team he is one of the top runners, and he is to be congratulated on his second place in the

The Green Dragon

Dunelm Run. I look forward to an even better season next year." For the next three years, the Dunelmian run was won by an International athlete at school called Edwin James. I was second to him once at the 10 mile distance, but he was in a different league.

We used to get up early mornings to tend the school's highland cattle with Ed Halford, Edwin James and Rev. Fernyhough, and at an annual 'cattle exhibition' I led a black bull called Hamish. Ed invited me to the society dinner and it was a grand occasion indeed, with bagpipes, Scottish dancing and much revelry from all angles.

I met Esther Aspinall at the City trials for cross-country. The girls set off first, then the boys. I started to overtake and we started to chat en route. Then weeks later we met by chance in Klute nightclub one Saturday night and exchanged phone numbers. She attended Durham Johnston school and I attended Durham school, both in the same age group. We met up several times but we didn't work out for long. One factor was Dan Downing who left my school after GCSEs, switched to Durham Johnston, and had something to do with us splitting up.

It was around this age that I started to go out into town at weekends. I can remember pubs like 'The Coach and Eight', 'Swan and Three Cygnets', 'The Dun Cow', 'The Duke of Wellington', and our regular nightclub 'Klute'. I was often invited to spend nights at Rupert Ellis's house. The Ellises were a big family and kept a detailed guest book to keep track of their visitors. My entries into that visitors' book were off the wall in some respects because my head was beginning to go off around this age. I had asked Megan Ellis, Rupert's sister, if she would go out with me but got rejected. She preferred the rugby players. Rupert played trumpet with excellence, Barney (elder brother) played flute and piano magnificently, and Megan could sing like a diva.

Every year there was a 'House song competition'. Bungites' songs over the years included: Swing Low Sweet Chariot,

Rawhide, Yesterday (arranged by Rupert and myself), and Dedicated Follower of Fashion (The Kinks). The Part-song component was a small group. Anthony Cleeve was a year older than me and left school at 16. He could sing properly, 'Cleevage'! With songs ranging from 'Goodnight, Sweetheart', 'In the Jungle the Lion Sleeps Tonight' to 'Lollipop' - Chris Cartner, Rupert Ellis, Richard Gatland, Howell Wong and myself were also involved in the house part song. Richard once commented that I seemed "cool as a cucumber" before going on stage. Howell Wong was conductor for the main song group in his last year and was also a 3rd degree blackbelt in taekwondo. He had been coaching me for a year or so and got me to 'green tag' level with WTF taekwondo (World Taekwondo Federation), which involved sparring, fitness and patterns. Other students learning the martial art at the time were Leo Hui, Gareth Blackbird, Adam Brown, and David Curry. Master Dave Jordan (5th Dan) was called in to the school to adjudicate as we were tested. Howell used to joke around but he could seriously move well when required. He was also on the school rowing team, coxless fours with Richard Gatland, Andrew Bayles, and Alex Lowrie.

At the end of every autumn term in December, before the Christmas holidays, we had the school Christmas dinner, followed by house entertainments back in all our houses – School, Poole, Caffinites, Langley, Ferens, and Pimlico. At School house, our final end of year farewell was to all link arms and hands right the way up the 3 floor stairwell and sing the school anthem 'Floreat Dunelmia', and then Auld Lang Syne (ahead of schedule). This usually raised the roof for a few minutes!

One birthday, the boys in my year, organised by Mark Nixon, arranged a fundraiser to pay for my return train ticket to York to spend my birthday weekend with Kerry Armitage, a friend whom I had met at the Joseph Rowntree festival one time in York. She went from York sixth form college to Durham University before signing up for work with Yorkshire Water.

The Green Dragon

This was one year before I started to go out with Hannah Teale, also of York Sixth Form College.

In the year's new dormitory I pinned up surreal posters and began to experiment with cannabis on occasion. One time Luke and myself climbed out of the dorm after lights out onto the roof enclosure and shared a joint. Reetesh had always made a point of saying 'no' to any smoking, and went on to an American University where smoking and drinking were completely banned. He used to wonder what his future wife was doing now, and he and his brother Rahul were both set to enter the hotel industry later, as their father owned a chain of Hong Kong hotels. Reetesh was a friend whilst we were at Durham school. I smoked my first cigarette by the banks of the River Wear, with a group of colleagues including Matthew Johnson (nicknamed 'Biddy' – he also did GCSE music and played flute).

My 16th birthday was celebrated in The Rose and Crown pub at home in Beadlam/Nawton with some school friends, though we claimed it was my 18th for legal purposes, and passed it off. I remember Mark Nixon, Reetesh Saraf, Andrew Malone, Rupert Ellis and Matthew Johnson all with me at that time. Our paths drifted apart within a year, though.

At various parties and festivals in the holidays, my brother Jonny introduced me to his circle of hippy friends and I would participate in smoking a joint if it was passed to me. One time I danced wildly in the crowd and ripped the microphone stand from the stage causing much consternation with others. I kept dancing and eventually others joined in as well. Jonny drove a motorbike and gave me a lift home afterwards late at night.

In the summer immediately following my GCSEs I worked as a haybailer at the Trevelyans' farm in Spaunton, North Yorkshire. Philip and Nelly were friends of my parents and had two sons and a daughter: Jack, Matthew, and Suzanna. That summer I also worked as a waiter at The Pheasant Inn, Harome, N Yorks. Unfortunately, my dearest brother Jonny offered me LSD and I accepted. I took half a tab one night when I should have been watching the Wimbledon tennis on telly. That affected me long term. The pair of us were up through the night hallucinating and giggling at everything. Ben Scott learnt of the incident at work the next morning. I had been up all night tripping, age 16. This was three years after Andre Agassi had won the championship title.

Soon after making the choice to stay on at Durham school I turned 17. Having been on a York music course in the holidays, I had started to 'go out' with the beautiful Yorkie Hannah Teale. We were in completely different cities the whole time, seeing each other at weekends only. We had a musical connection, having been brought up to play a stringed instrument. Hannah played cello, and I played viola. We were both young and enjoyed similar interests, although in fairness our relationship was indeed 'puppy love' and I was getting quite messed up in my own mind at times throughout our year together. I can remember hero-worshipping Forrest Gump when the movie came out in 1996. This probably put Hannah onto her closer college friends, whilst I was simultaneously starting to struggle spiritually searching for answers about the eternal, ie 'is there a God?' I can't remember when or how, but at some point I must have concluded that there is a God, because I asked the Reverend Fernyough if he would baptise and confirm me that year. Several witnesses came to the baptism including David Lascelles, Ed Halford, and Michael Ellis. There were times it seemed to me that God and the devil were battling for my soul.

A beautiful moment when it felt like I had found God was on top of a snow-capped mountain in Scotland, on an adventure week to Crianlarich with Mr Burgess, Gareth Jones, Alex Lowrie, Andrew Johnson, Colin Murray, Gareth's dad, Edward somebody, Jenny Growcott, and Mr Cook. We had been dividing the week into mountain-biking, canoeing, abseiling/rock climbing, bothying/mountaineering which involved a 4 am start to the day, to discover that we had been sharing the cabin with some rodents who ate some essential provisions overnight. I remember Andrew Johnson shouting that a rat had nibbled his face in the night. I went outside to meditate on a rock with

Gareth Jones and sing 'Bohemian Rhapsody'. We were walking non-stop until about 7pm that evening covering 3 Johnson mountains and 3 Murray mountains in between, covered in rocky snow and ice. We had to use crampons and pick axes. When we got to the car park the minibus was the most welcome sight ever, back to civilisation.

In the Upper sixth year I spoke at The Heretics Society about the problems of having so many separate languages. I proposed Esperanto as a common second language, presenting financial and time implications about translations. They needed more about cultural implications so 'burnt' me as a heretic, convinced that English will be the only satisfactory international language.

One time there was a Lascelles party at their home. At some point in the proceedings I was asked to find some smokes for them from the next door neighbours, so I walked with Andrew Malone to knock on the door. They were surprised by the request, but on hearing it to be a party decided to bob along for themselves to join in. As far as I can remember they did in fact bring some smokes for David to buy.

In terms of subjects, I had chosen to study A-levels in Music, Biology, French, and General Studies. My sixth form experience was largely music-oriented, taking part in Orchestras – school, Northern Junior Philharmonic Orchestra (Ripon NJPO 1996), and Young Sinfonia (Newcastle 1996/97), I had some viola ambitions at the time despite the fact that girls were entering in the sixth form. I just wanted to focus on my music. Confirmed and baptised age 17 with a belief in God, my spiritual struggle had begun. Hannah had left me for somebody else, following a summer orchestral course in Durham. I remember walking for miles in a state of hurt and confusion.

Xenophon Kelsey's 'Vacation Chamber Orchestra' in the North Yorkshire/Dales region provided an outlet for these musical notions. I met Gary Matthewman (trumpet and piano) who in later years became an international concert pianist. In Scarborough, over the years, I twice saw him play a piano concerto – Grieg and then Mozart. Also brightly talented were John, Paul, and Neville (violin/viola), and Stephen Provine (violin leader/piano) who got into Harvard University, plus many other bright young, talented people with whom I played games amongst the girls and boys. But I had started to get ill mentally by now, probably owing to the LSD, cannabis and magic mushrooms I had once taken at a Brandsby house party, at the then home of Lossinder Holland aka 'Lossie', one of Jonny's friends, where they were mostly hippy people into experimental drugs. I got invited along to a few of their parties/festivals, and without much ado I went and took part in the proceedings.

There were parties at the Ellis' home of Rupert, Barney, Megan, mum Sue (social worker), and dad Bill (gynaecologist). Rupert drove us in a car every Sunday to Orchestra in Newcastle (Young Sinfonia). I played for a year before I felt too stressed out and lost all interest in the viola. Kirsten Stewart and Jessica Howard from Newcastle both expressed an interest in me at some point. I did like them but my head was getting messed up so couldn't deal with it all.

I stayed with Michael Ellis once a week for another orchestral rehearsal. He smoked a lot and liked to hang out with John Pratt (French Horn), who plays professionally today with the Opera North Orchestra. My mother and I went to watch a Jose Carreras/Kiri te Kanawa opera concert at the opening of Scarborough's Open Air Theatre (July 2010), and John Pratt was then playing French Horn. He was also a proficient viola player! Michael and John could talk for hours about anything. Mark Blenkiron lived just up the road. Myself and others referred to his impressively advanced piano style as 'Blenking'. Mark had previously played chess for England, was a computer expert and tried for Cambridge, but got to Edinburgh University instead. We once went out on a training run together but he was no athlete.

In athletics, I was miraculously school captain and won the senior Kingston run, and came 2nd to Edwin James in the Dunelmian 10 miles as previously mentioned. He was a

Nationals standard runner. Hannah Teale and Rupert Ellis cheered me on from the sidelines. Another time I ran a 5 mile fun run in York with my brother Chris. We dressed up as hippies and he proceeded to juggle all the way round the course, causing such comments as "Oi, matey don't drop your balls!" I dated Hannah for a year having met on the Junior Yorchestra circuit. In truth I preferred Juliet Bedford but never got her. Hannah eventually dumped me for somebody else. I also tried to see somebody else – Alex Hanky, but that fell through very quickly. Alex was on my music course and played piano, violin, clarinet and sang well. She ended up attending a musical conservatoire. On a vacation Northern Junior Philharmonic Orchestral (NJPO) course, I played viola badly one time only. The auditions were a big event, but I got in on account of viola players being a rarer breed. We gave a concert in Ripon cathedral as part of an International Festival in 1996. At that time, although offered lessons on guitar by Sue Elm, I had no interest in learning that instrument until years later.

All I wanted to do was practice viola and piano. A small group of us formed a barbershop singing group which we called 'The Revellers'. That was Rupert's idea. Chris Cartner, Gareth Jones, Philip Osbourne, Michael Ellis, Rupert Ellis and myself. Matthew Courtney took my place when I couldn't cope anymore. One time I broke down in the dinner hall at Rupert. I shouted. He had interrupted an Athletics club dinner calling me to singing rehearsal. I nearly punched him; really felt like it, but didn't. Matthew was a good friend whilst I was at Durham – keen rugby player, National Youth Choir, sharp debating skills, actor and Head of Poole House. Matthew was deputy Head of School the year after I left, but Christopher Hilton of Langley just got the honour. Today, Chris is a practising psychiatric Doctor, based near Paddington in London.

That year the school choir went on a day trip to Blackpool, courtesy of Roger Muttit, the new Music Director. All I remember about this is trying to hit it off with Emma Thickness, walking on the beach topless with Matthew Courtney, and him buying me five straight rides on the Pepsi Max ride. We took pride in showing off our splendid pectorals to all the girls. Youth of Britain shout it out loud "I've got splendid pectorals and I'm proud!" (Harry Enfield).

My heart sank ten years later when I read in the school Dunelmian magazine that Matt had died tragically aged 26. I found out from Chris on Facebook that he had fallen from a great height in London's Tate Modern Art Gallery. An absolute tragedy, but I always remember Matthew for being the best. Three other school-boy deaths during my time at Durham were the heartbreaking cases of Philip Scorer, Richard Cawthorn, and David Reay. Philip was playing football at home, ran out of his drive into the road to fetch the ball and got fatally struck by a car. Richard had been nominated to be next year's headboy of Caffinites house. He was on a moorland expedition and by the end of the walk complained of bad headaches. He told his doctor soon after returning, but a week later he had passed away at 17. I am not sure about the cause of the headaches. David Reay suffered leukaemia and after a long and painful struggle, he passed away in hospital also aged 17.

Two teaching heads of department arranged a continental trip. Mr Muttit and Mr Crook organised a French/Music school trip to Paris involving music, choir, and plenty of French. I remember some special recitals by Dylan Pugh (cello) who lost his mother when he was 17, Robert Ainsley (conductor/organ), Leon Wang (violin), Roger Muttit (Director), and Mr Mark Mawhinney (assistant). Robert won the school music competition, the 'Chadeyron' more than once, and I was lucky to take part in my final year on piano and viola. In Paris we struggled with the Metro system and I visited Jim Morrison's (The Doors) grave in Paris with Simon Shaw, Robert English, and Diccon Humphrey. Diccon was seeing Liberty Kidd in sixth form. She was a stunning blonde, looking to pursue an acting dream after school. They were once found taped up together in the engineering room.

My French class that year included Paul Watson, Galine Cleary, Bill Murray, Rupert Ellis, Simon Reay, Mark Nixon, Andrew

Bayles (Headboy) et al. During the visit Mr Crook gave each student 10 euros to spend. We visited Sacre Coeur, Notre Dame, Le Louvre, Eiffel Tower, L'Arc de Triomphe and Les Invalides, and tried French crêpes. Will Murray and Philip Osbourne spent some time with me during this trip. Will was a fantastic tenor singer, and Philip an Oxbridge scholar. Will had a lead role in the school musical 'Godspell' for which I auditioned but got rejected. I went to all three nights when the time came to watch. Really, I just fancied Megan Ellis and wanted to be together with her. She also had a lead role in the musical. When I asked her out she told me that she wasn't interested in boys. However, I was invited to her 18th birthday ball at Newcastle's Tuxedo Royale nightclub on a boat, on the river Tyne. I dressed up as did we all, and danced a lot that night.

Back at Durham, one Sunday evening in the regular chapel service I nearly fainted so got walked to san for the night. I had started to write my Biology essays in multi coloured pens. Mr Burgess commented on this habit. Mrs Evans used to make jokes about this and the style of my writing as well. My Biology class for A-levels included Galine Cleary, Alistair Lowe, Jessica Bell, Alex Hazel, Anne Everett, Paul Watson, Andrew Bayles, Philip Osbourne (Cavemen speech at debate), Alex Lowrie, et al.

Every week there was a sixth form lecture for the senior year to attend and one time it was about Esperanto given by my Dad. He had been teaching the language as a keen advocate for years, and had taught me Esperanto since the Terrington years. Plus there were weekly lessons in the school library in a small group including the Librarian (Mrs Watkins), David Curry, Jan Trutschler (a German), Reetesh Saraf, myself, and occasionally others, too.

Once, in the library, whilst perusing the shelves, I spotted a library book called "Unlimited Power" by Anthony Robbins. Although at the time I couldn't make head or tail of it – too heavy for my simple mind – I read it properly 10 years later and attended three of his world famous seminars in London 2006/07 (aged 27/28) which provided some further education for me.

In my Upper sixth year, aged 18, all my essays were now written in plain blue ink. When I was awarded an A grade for a music essay I felt duly rewarded. My music class included Michael Ellis (clarinet), Joe Cragg James (violin), Rachel Snaith (saxophone), Rupert Ellis (trumpet), Alex Hanky (piano/clarinet), and myself (viola).

I had hoped to become Head Boy by this point, but my head was all over the place and I was quite messed up in fact, so never even got noticed throughout my sixth form experience. My sporting athletics days seemed to be over, debating skills were atrocious, heretics society talked of Esperanto – most voted against, no Durham girlfriend, people lost all interest in me. I wasn't listed for either CCF or Community Voluntary work. Maybe I should have gone to York sixth form instead? I reckon that Durham forgot I was even there by the time I had finished at the school. My last year was lonely and people were saying I was a weirdo. Tristan Prosser once set me up to make it sound like I was breaking into store rooms underneath the theatre. People believed him on account of being a 1st XV rugby player and later, captain.

One time I was called upon to play in the 4th XV rugby team. I had to carry a crate of water 1.5 miles to the pitch before the match and only just made it before the starting whistle blew.

Mr Dias remained interested and supportive in my endeavours, though. Towards the end of every summer term, there were the Annual House Barbecues. At School House we were blessed with Mr Hirsch, Mr Newell, Mr Hind, and Mr Zafer who did the New Zealand Haka Maori style one year. I asked Mr Dias to play guitar for us, and he promptly sang Sloop John B by The Beach Boys. Meanwhile Kenneth Shepherd was organising a giant-sized newspaper rizla/cigar-type smoke to be passed round the bonfire. I didn't go for that though. Ken was the 1st XV rugby captain that year, having stayed on an extra year to complete his work.

In the study rooms I remember talking with Michael Cannon, who loved cricket, Takashi Hirano from Asia, and Florian Wolkner from Germany (whom I met the following summer in his home town of Dortmund during an inter-railing expedition). One time I walked Michael's sister, Amanda Cannon, home from the pub after a night out. She was seeing Gareth Blackbird at the time. In the year 2010, we remet on Facebook and exchanged a few words once again. I once shared a study room with Fraser Watts from Scotland who was into cricket in a big way. He ended up with the girl I wanted to invite to the end of year ball, though.

On a positive note, my post-school plans involved fundraising for a 3 month expedition to Indonesia. In order to raise funds I organised a 12 hour sponsored concert involving 18 musicians at school. Annabel Trapp from York was considering coming to the school to play in the event! This event raised approximately £150 but Chris Cartner and Gareth Jones pretended to run away with the money at the end of the day. They gave it back to me, though, which mattered to me. There were prizes for best performance, most original performance, most appearances made, and largest donation received. Sponsored by Boots, HMV, and Oddbins wine I got some prizes together. However, I never made it to Indonesia – I took ill at home (which is a story for subsequent chapters) and forwarded the funds to Trekforce, to the International Scientific Support Trust. The funds went to Trekforce scientific researchers, along with £50 from a sponsored bungee jump.

Results day at Durham school involved a drop-off, walk to board, check results – Biology (B), General Studies (B), French (C), Music (C), pizza hut with dad, then a group gathering at the Coach and Eight pub in town, with many members of my year there: Luke Hunter Patterson (played late night ninjas in Lower V once), Joe Cragg James, Ian Laidler, Chris Wilde (whose 18th birthday was a massive party at his dad's greyhound racing stadium near Sunderland), Alistair Lowe (Head of house), Alex Hazel (his then girlfriend) and Galine Cleary whom he married in subsequent years. I then took a walk by the river Wear all the way to the Ellis' house and there they were holding a final leaving party for Rupert and friends. I was invited so appreciated having somewhere to go.

I always enjoyed singing in Durham cathedral with the school choir when the time came, and walking back by the River Wear afterwards. Quite often I would catch a train from Durham to Thirsk at the weekend, to go home. Then back again Sunday night. There were others making the same journey, including John Mosey and a girl called Hannah. I didn't mind the travelling as it gave me time to think.

When I left Durham School, that was it for school. I dreamt of going to Oxford University, but in reality was way, way off from that sort of thing. I never had the grades for a start. I had been offered a place at the Royal Holloway University in London to read French and Music. I changed my mind and decided that I wanted to read French and Italian to impress the girls. It didn't happen. I was on a GAP year intending to firstly travel to Indonesia on a Trekforce expedition, then go ahead as planned. However, the story that unfolds is something that I hadn't planned; a decade of change.

Chapter Three
Blind Ambition

Have you ever dreamed of a life by the Mediterranean, soaking in the sun and strolling along the promenades? Speculating on the warm sunshine and tranquil, clear blue sea? I have.

During my time at Durham School sixth form I began to formulate an itinerary for a month's trip around Europe in the summer immediately following my A-levels. Having asked around to see who might be interested to join me there were two of us who had agreed to travel together. My colleague, Alex Lowrie, was also a Biology student, something of a gymnast, and a technician for plays and musicals, operating the sound and lighting. Four other students had initially been interested to come, but opted to go to Tenerife in a group, instead, to celebrate their summer there.

We were 18 years old. School had finished. What could be better than a month's untrammelled freedom travelling round Europe to find our feet in the big world?

We initially visited Newcastle railway station to purchase our 'freedom passes' for which the whole of Europe was divided into zones. We selected a ticket to cover one month's travel in France, Holland, Germany, and Denmark. This cost just less than £500, for which I made use of some inheritance money. I had also recently opened a bank account with Natwest and they gave me a Visa card and a Mastercard to travel with £1,000 credit.

Our selected date to arrive in Calais, France, was Tuesday 8th July. Alex was arranging a lift with some colleagues to get us there. As it happens, Alex lived on a farm near Durham city, and I lived near York, so we would have to co-ordinate the meeting place. The weekend before, I had been in York with a friend, Juliet Bedford, who had seen me off at York station on the way to Caistor to see another school friend, Andy Millson, who had something of a little farewell celebration for me in the local area with others.

I had arranged to meet Alex and minibus at Doncaster MoatHouse Hotel on Tuesday lunchtime. So, accordingly, Andy dropped me off at Caistor station and I went to Doncaster to wait. Hours later the minibus arrived full of a hardy bunch of…..bootleggers! They were going to acquire whisky and cigarettes on the continent and sell them back in the UK for a profit. Alex and myself sat fairly quietly during the lift to Dover. They were raucous!

At Dover we were bought our ferry tickets for Calais, and got on the ferry. There we were given £20 and instructed to buy two bottles of whisky each. This would have resulted in approximately 14 bottles of whisky for them, but duty free regulations disallowed the second bottle, so they ended up with just seven bottles. We sat in the lounge and walked about on deck during the journey.

At the Calais ferry port we were unceremoniously dumped with rucksacks and bade "bon voyage". So we were left with a long walk into Calais town from the port. We walked, arriving at the campsite at around 2am, fairly tired already on day one. Here we set up tent and camped out. Waking around 9am the next morning for breakfast, our time on the continent had thus begun.

We walked into the town centre and went in search of an ATM and the railway station. Here we got our first taste of French francs (at the time). With our pockets loaded up we then sat at a bistro table eating baguettes and drinking some Kronenbourg. We decided to get on with the trip and got on a train to Amiens. Here we looked around for a couple of hours and on the same day travelled to Paris.

As we had arranged previously, we had strapped rollerblades to our rucksacks; one pair each. These were ideally to be used on the Mediterranean promenades, but we soon discovered an area near the Youth Hostel (Paris Arpajon) on the outskirts of the city, where we could explore on the blades. Getting to the hostel was a challenge in itself, crossing the city on busy local metro trains, but we made it and pitched the tent in the garden for one night only. The whole trip was a whistle stop tour – a night here, a night there. In the area where we were on roller-blades, we tried to enter a shop to buy a drink, but the shopkeeper got fairly angry at us. "Zut, alors! Pas ici messieurs!" he said, or words to that effect.

We returned to camp, having explored the vicinity, and made something to eat. Alex informed me of his ambition to learn harmonica and promptly whipped out a "tin sandwich" to play for a while. He was just beginning.

In the morning we were rudely awoken by early morning road works just next to the hostel, round about 7am. We decided to get up and make headway for the day. We were going to Lyon, France's industrial third city. Here I taught Alex how to juggle and we discovered a pretty cool music shop. I bought a Myron Waldren album to take home (jazz saxophone, piano and drum trio). We only stayed until the evening. Here we caught the train to go to St Etienne.

At St Etienne the campsite was really inconvenient. It involved walking up a 1½ mile steep hill with rucksacks on. We met two Dutch girls on the campsite and chatted for a while. Then into town for something to eat. Back down the hill! On the search for a McDonalds we were misdirected by a devious young Frenchman and ended up going to a pizzeria. "Chez McDo's s'il vous-plait?" Maybe he was a joker at heart. Very funny!

Back up the hill at night to the tent. We had contacted my French exchange family to ask if we could call in for a few days. They didn't seem to mind. The LeFranc family lived on a Limousin cattle farm near Chateauroux, in the centre of France 100km north of Limoges. Luc and Elizabeth were parents to Thomas (farm hand, now married), Edouard (cellist and law student), Guillaume (tennis player and pianist), and Charles (saxophonist and youngest brother). We caught the 5am train on

Saturday July 12th from St Etienne – Lyon – Clermont Ferrand – Chateauroux, arriving at about 2pm. At the station I phoned up and we were given a lift to the farm that afternoon. They had a swimming pool, tennis court and basketball court on the farm, with a quad bike, so plenty to do during our stay. We were roped into fruit-picking for a neighbour. My French was reasonable so I managed to talk to the others from time to time. Alex enjoyed the farm, being brought up in that kind of environment. Their dog moulted outside our tent one evening so we woke up to a massive pile of fur on the lawn. Alex had assisted the moulting process a little, to be fair. The LeFrancs were extremely hospitable towards us and a lot of fun, too.

After two nights here we caught the train from Chateauroux to Nice via Verzon and Lyon. Back home, friends of the family, the Beggs (David, Margaret, Catriona and friend) had agreed to let us stay with them on a campsite in Valbonne, near Nice. They owned a static caravan, we had a tent, but they let us eat with them and play cards and other games. One night a neighbour, whom I had met in the swimming pool earlier on, came home late. I went to talk to them and it turned out that she had been in a car crash that day. So we soberly drank some water and took time to recover. Her sister was driving and broke her collar bone. She knew an acquaintance from Durham sixth form – Tim Cuthbertson – and we talked about him for a while. I believe he went into the army after school.

Round about this time in the UK it was Juliet Bedford's 18th birthday. She had very kindly invited me to be there. I had very thoughtlessly turned her down in favour of my travels. Around the 15th July I made a phone call. She seemed pleased to hear from me. Maybe I should have come back home for this? A call from Nice. Not all that bad I hope!

The most usual food we ate on the trains was baguette chunks with jam, cold meat, cheese, or chocolate spread on them. We once invented the world's worst pasta supper with pasta twirls, beef oxo gravy and chocolate spread. Utterly disgusting! But we learnt.

The Green Dragon

Now we had made it to the Mediterranean at last after all that thought over the last two years. We took our roller-blading skills onto the promenade but were rapidly overtaken by a venerable pensioner going backwards on one foot slaloming in between coke cans. We were truly humbled. There were plenty of pedestrians to weave amongst.

In the evenings, David Begg treated us all to restaurant meals, and we met a friend of theirs who seemed offended by my mannerisms. Can't remember names, but he still offered me a beer anyway with everyone else. Catriona's friend Leona got on really well with Alex. We got back late to camp and it was warm enough to literally sleep under the stars, so I did.

The next morning I paid a visit to the reception to buy postcards and stamps. Here I managed to muster enough French to flirt with the receptionist. That was pretty cool. She ended up giving us a lift to the bus station rather than have us walk five miles along the road. We passed through Cannes (film festival not on at this time), Marseilles (known for a criminal underworld), and headed West to Bordeaux on Thursday, July 17th.

The purpose of this move was to meet a group of young Germans who were camping on the Atlantic Coast in 'Camping Municipal du Gurpe'. They had previously attended Durham sixth form and given us their dates of arrival here. Their names were: Max, Anka, Lisa, Philip, Sarah, and Florian. We had to catch a bus for 10km from central Bordeaux and then roller-blade 5km with rucksacks on, guessing the way to the coastal campsite.

Ironically the Brits and Germans met once again on the shores of France. This time in friendly circumstances. They made us all a huge bucket of pasta and we exchanged tales thus far. On the beach Alex and I bought body-boards and caught some waves. Also sun-bathed a little. In the evenings people lit bonfires on the beach and Philip had brought his guitar so sang some German pop to us all. Unlike the calm Mediterranean with pebbled beaches, here there were waves and sand. On the beaches were a lot of former WW2 bunkers. People generally clambered on top of them and sat in groups talking. We all did, with guitar music too.

Quite appropriately, having met the Germans here, our next stop was to be Germany itself. We needed to return to Bordeaux station and travel north to Paris, and then have a complete change – East and South to Munich, Bavaria, Germany. This involved an overnight journey. We sat separately and my neighbour got off at Ulm in the early hours. At Gare de L'Est, Paris, there were armed guards patrolling the station so everyone felt a bit wary of their business there.

In Munich we had agreed to stay with the Kuetgen family. Erik had been a personal friend in the sixth form, at Durham. We stayed there for five nights. Once there, we travelled by bike and on foot. Erik showed us the cultural sights of Munich…the Chinese Tower in the English Garden, the TV tower, Munich city museum, the Frauenkirche and late one night I made a personal exploration into 'Kunst-park Ost' a set of industrial warehouses converted into music halls ranging from Rap and Hip-Hop, to R'n'B, to Rock and Heavy Metal. I danced the night away to some Hip Hop music and missed the last train home at 2am so was stuck at the station until 5am. I cycled back to the Kuetgen's house by 6.30am. Erik and Alex were almost getting up already for a day's cycling venture.

Although they were on the list, we never made it to the Bavarian film studios. Erik took us to a breakfast café and treated us to a true Bavarian 'Weissbier' breakfast of boiled sausage, sweet mustard, and a pint of white German beer. This was in fact delicious. Alex and I decided to split up for two days and meet again at Berlin station at 12noon Monday, July 28th. We had been in close company for almost three weeks by now so needed a break. We said thankyou and goodbye to the Kuetgens after a further day trip to mad King Ludwig's eccentric castle (Neuschwannstein Schloss). My German language was minimal, but we were blessed by the Kuetgens' grasp of English.

The Green Dragon

I travelled alone to Heidelberg and Hannover, staying in Youth Hostels and walking about town for a while. Not much to report from these trips. So, on the Monday, Alex and I met once again at Berlin station at noon. We walked about the city, and took in some culture – the Brandenburg Gate, the Kaiser Wilhelm memorial church (left as a monument to WW2 with, still today, the steeple blown in half by bombers), the Berlin TV mast (99 feet taller than the Eiffel Tower!), and the zoo. We sampled 'Berlin Weisse' a type of beer that comes with either red or green syrup. This drink is unique to Berlin. Then later that day, being young and foolish, we had both agreed to head to Holland, to Amsterdam and sample its famed culture.

In Amsterdam we stayed at a Youth Hostel for three nights. We went straight for the kill and found our way into a 'café' and placed an order from the 'menu'. Our stuff was all at the Arena youth hostel and we were in town looking for the group of Germans with whom to get stoned on the canals of Amsterdam. Sure enough, we located their hostel and left a message on the board. We had a reply within 5 hours so met up that evening and spent the night sitting on a barge smoking 'Black Gold' in a joint being passed around. That seemed really awesome at the time. Maybe it was disaffecting, though, after all.

We toured the cycler's city on foot, bearing witness to slopey buildings by the canals, and museums, and I even dyed my hair yellow. Only it turned out more pale green at the time. Back at the Arena hostel we talked to some others and made our plans for the next step. By this point Alex knew that he had to return home early to help his father on the farm, so we had only a few more days together. On the train to Dortmund we hid the resin in the rucksack framework. We met Florian Wolkner at Dortmund station and he welcomed us to their family for three nights.

My first choice of activity was to go the whole hog and peroxide my hair blonde-white. It was a shock at first for a day or two. The Wolkners lived in a big house and had big-wig important family connections in the world of German business. One night they held a party and many people were there. In a side room were the youngsters, and in the main room the Directors, Managers and senior figures. We unveiled the resin from the rucksack and passed it round. This time it got to my head – I had a whiteout. One of Florian's friends was the 1995 European kickboxing champion and on recovering we found we were all outside. I started dancing and mimicking Taekwondo patterns, everyone derived mirth from this.

Florian dumped us at Dortmund station on Sunday, August 3rd. Alex was headed back home to the farm, I was due to remain travelling for one more week. That was the last I saw of Alex until we got our A-level results later that month back in Durham.

I had one more family to visit in Hannover – the Baums. Robin and Sonia had both been students in Durham sixth form. Sonia and I used to go running together. Robin was by now an up-and-coming politician and soldier. He drove a Mercedes Benz at the age of 19!

On the way to Hannover I stopped at Koln for the afternoon. Here I toured the cathedral, walked by the river Rhine, and witnessed a xylophone player playing Khachaturian's 'Sabre Dance' – blindfolded! Mythology has it that Koln was once subject to a devastating fireball.

Then on to Hannover and the Baum family. Sonia kept a pet ferret and two dogs. She was a superb pianist and dreamed of becoming a famous author later on. She went to Bonn University. Together we visited a restaurant and an ice-cream parlour. We walked by a lake on a cool evening. But, unfortunately the trip to Amsterdam was beginning to take its toll.

Yet again I was blessed with the family's knowledge of English. I would have been stumped if it had come to speaking in German.

The Green Dragon

The next day I went solo to Hamburg and walked up the Reeperbahn for fun. Also, I sat by the docks for a while and bought my brothers some souvenirs. Then back to Hannover. The last breakfast was sitting out on the patio in the early morning, eating German breads, cold meats, salami and yogurt with fruit with Sonia. Then I was given a lift to the station and headed to Calais, via Paris. After another overnight train journey in a small cabin I returned home.

All in all, I found the trip Inter-railing entertaining, educational, fun, zany, crazed, inspiring and sociable. Although the travelling itself was maybe a little uncomfortable, I would have liked to get to Denmark or Spain. Maybe some other time? We were lucky to have so many contacts to stay with, otherwise there would have been much more camping and Youth Hostelling. I am glad to have had the opportunity to do this as an eighteen year old. My life did change because of the trip, maybe not exactly the way I would have liked, but it changed.

An Inter-railing, European bonanza and an eye-opener! With God's goodness of grace, hopefully there would be chance to travel the world again one day!

Back home in the caravan where I lived then at my parents' house, I wrote a ten year plan. I came up with everything I would like to do and achieve by the age of 30. Precious little actually went according to plan. Ranging from becoming a 3rd degree black belt taekwondo athlete with a shot at the Olympic Games Gold medal, to a political thought – become Prime Minister; then financially – to become a millionaire by the age of 30, to musically – become a world famous singer/songwriter/conductor/artist/concert pianist, etc, to run the London marathon, and of course to get married with family round about age 30. I had many respectable notions about what I would like to do with my life after school. At one point, all I wanted to do was to be known as a viola player and the delusion was to go play in the Berlin Philharmonic Orchestra, but in reality, I struggled to keep up with the youth orchestras I had already played in.

When I lived in the caravan, I was friends with Charles Dale of Kirkbymoorside. He was learning Bass guitar, training as a DJ, and joined the Jesus army. I used to knock on his window to see if he was doing much at the time. He knew some guy called Mario who later went on to become a millionaire in business. Charlie, as he prefers to be known to friends, joined a Production management team for the Hovingham quarry and has been working with them for many years, making a mint. We used to go driving with Tim to random places, just to get away from our homes for a while. My poor head had started to go elsewhere round about this time, but we listened to music and that was all until August 2010 when Tim reintroduced us at Scarborough Blues club, and then, on Facebook. He told me not to be a stranger any more and keep in touch. Charlie bought a copy of my book, Plan 103f, when we met again.

At the end of 1997, my first steps into the big bad world were taken. Whilst learning to drive in Malton with Barry Fothergill, I studied for grade 8 piano at Ampleforth College (taught by David Bowman), attended taekwondo classes in Burton Stone Lane sports hall, York, and worked in the local BATA garage in Helmsley as a Forecourt/shop assistant, and washed pots in the Star Inn, Harome, but shortly got sacked from both jobs within a three month period. As it transpired, this was as close to a working career as I would ever get in my life. I was a dreamer, so found it hard to focus on the mundanities at hand. In December 1997 I took and passed my practical driving test in Malton, and theory in York. Somehow I passed both first time round and was granted my driving licence. The taekwondo lasted less than a year. I got into a shouting match with the instructor Fiona Brown (4th Dan) and felt too embarrassed to return to the dojo, so gave my uniform back again.

At the same time I was taking piano lessons with David Bowman at Ampleforth College for a Grade 8 examination, at the age of 19. Between the two of us I managed to acquire a Distinction at the end of 1997, having attempted the exam and failed twice previously whilst at Durham. Third time lucky! I played Beethoven's sonata in F# major, JS Bach's Prelude and Fugue in

The Green Dragon

F# major, and three dances by Shostakovich. As my parents had both taught music there for over two decades it seemed right to get a result like that. At Durham School I had twice failed the exam with Debussy's Serenade of the Doll, Scarlatti's Study in Em, and Haydn Sonata in Em. So, new place, new pieces – third time lucky!

For my 19th birthday I had four tickets for a 'Blur' pop concert at Hull Arena. Somehow I got my old school friend Andy Milson to come from Loughborough with a new friend, and my Terrington Hall crush, Michelle Wood, agreed to attend, with me driving. I collected her from her home in Bulmer on the afternoon then drove to Hull to meet Andy and friend at McDonalds prior to attending the gig. Tickets cost £15 each, so thanks to Mum and Dad for paying as a birthday gift.

The concert was awesome, wildly exciting and long anticipated. We danced and sang in the crowd. The Blur album, Parklife, had been huge during my GCSE year 1995. Eventually the group, with Damon Albarn singing - and co, calmed down again and "let us" go home. Michelle and I said 'bye to Andy and friend then we set off for the 1½ hour drive home again. About midnight I dropped Michelle off at her home and made my way alone in the car. The roads were icy and cold at this hour and my judgement of Bulmer bank proved imperfect. I skidded off the road over a gravel heap and into a road sign at the top corner of the hill. The car wouldn't start again so I proceeded to dig at the gravel with a hub cap. I had actually been singing whilst driving, so this incident was entirely my own fault. Could have been worse.

A passerby at about 2am, who was driving, offered me a lift home. His story was that he was a depressed banker having a family crisis and needed time to think things through so got in his car and drove everywhere all night through. I got back home to Beadlam by 3am and expected a furious dad. He had lent me his car on trust after all. Instead, on the surface, he simply checked I was still alive, and asked specifically where the car was left for the breakdown truck to collect it the next day. This was to be one of my first major life lessons, of many.

Prior to getting the driving licence, and turning 19, I had another adventure after coming home from inter-railing. The Newcastle orchestra, Young Sinfonia, went on a concert tour to France. I was invited to be in the orchestra on viola. Our conductor was the young Ilan Volkov (himself just 19 years when he took the post), and the elected musical recitals were largely classical in style. We were scheduled to give concerts in French chateaux, churches, Limoges cathedral and other venues. Our bus ride was to be an overnight journey and we caught the ferry from Dover to Calais in the early hours. This event took place in August 1997, one week after I returned from my European travel adventures.

Names from that orchestral trip which I can recall now were Jake Spence (violin), Stephen Provine (violin-leader/piano), Stephen Moore (drums/percussion), Rupert Ellis (trumpet), Chris Cartner (oboe), Ilan Volkov (conductor), Jessica Howard (violin), Kirsten Stewart (violin), Daniel Hoare (viola), Yussef Albasri (viola), Rachel Hilton-Allen (Double Bass), Jamie Thomson (French Horn), John (violin), Ella Fearon (cello), Michael Ellis (clarinet), John Pratt (French Horn/viola), Vicki (violin), Jane (violin), et al. There were far more to remember worth talking about but my head was going crackapo at the time, so I struggle to remember more now.

We went on an excursion to a village called Oradour which had been obliterated by the Nazis during WW2 and it seemed surreal to look around the blown up and burnt-out buildings left behind. There was a memorial museum there, as well, listing all the residents who had been wiped out. It was said that some tried to escape into the surrounding woodlands but were shot down if seen running. My life suddenly seemed vulnerable from that moment on. I experienced a sense of mortality in Oradour that day. The village church had been used to hold the women and children, who were then burnt alive in the church, whilst the men were machine gunned down in the barns, or also burnt alive. I couldn't believe it.

I owe a debt of gratitude to the Young Sinfonia administration for giving me the opportunity to play with them for a year whilst finishing at Durham. The regular Sunday trips to Newcastle were an eye-opener and made me realise that life on the road was tougher than dreamed about. My head was already going off the rails by now, so unfortunately the last time I played a viola in an orchestra was December 1997, aged 19, at a Xenophon Kelsey Dales Chamber Orchestra vacation meeting, which was aimed at the young student population of North Yorkshire and elsewhere.

I attempted to play viola in the orchestra, but found myself lacking in ability and social competence, so soon packed it in, and my life became something I hadn't planned it to become. In the subsequent two years after leaving orchestral viola-playing behind, I attempted to become a concert pianist, practising for up to six hours a day at times. What I couldn't account for then was the mental breakdown that I was in fact experiencing. This breakdown affected all the family in a bad way.

In my head, I was dreaming of attending the Paris Conservatoire for a year to study piano. I set to learning Rachmaninov, Debussy, Bach, Mozart, Bartok and a lot of other music. Only, because my head wasn't functioning correctly, it was all just superficial noise and nothing was actually sinking into my memory. In effect, I was running away from everybody and everything. In June 1998 I put in for the Saltburn Music Festival on piano. My breakdown had led me to change my name to 'James Carlo Peter Owen'. My actual name was 'James Alexander Kershaw' aka 'Jamie'. When I went to Saltburn, Dad and Jonny came to listen. Geoffrey Emerson had written me a letter saying 'Good luck in Salzburg!' Somebody had been playing Chinese whispers or something. Salzburg I wish! There I played a Mozart Sonata in C, Rachmaninoff's Gm prelude, Debussy's Golliwogs Cakewalk, JS Bach's Prelude and Fugue in Bb major, and a couple of Bulgarian Dances by Bela Bartok. Around about that time I had been to Leeds College of Music for a trial audition, but because Nicki Isles was too busy to teach me I lost interest there. Also, I had an audition at the Royal Academy of Music in London with Vanessa Latarche. But because of my delinquency and delusions of going to Paris, I refused to take part in an English musical conservatoire. I was f#*%ed up! I now wish that I had seen straight and learnt jazz at Leeds, and classical at a London academy. In my head, because I had studied French and Music for A-level at Durham, the next step was both combined – a French music school, the Paris conservatoire. Alas, this was not to be, as were many of my youthful delusions not to be realised.

For quite some years I harboured the dream of writing a book, but not just any book – a million bestselling worldwide #1 book. Some years later, in 2006, round about the time that I was finishing at Hull University, I coined the idea for a title and a general idea for the sequence of events and characters involved. So round about April 2006 I began to write my first book, aged 27. Initially all I knew was that it was to be called 'Plan 103f', involving a select group of imaginary twenty-somethings living their dreams; ranging through Olympics, enterprise, romance, business, love, and friendship. Over a three year period I built on this idea and eventually completed writing a 256 page fiction/non-fiction novel. I applied to over 18 publishers and agents for publication approval but the offer I received was from Chipmunka Publishing in London - a Mental Health publishers. I contacted Jason Pegler (CEO) and he sent me the details. Having submitted the script for approval he sent me a contract which I signed within a week – June 2009 – and looked forwards to the paperback release in 2010. Paul Kirven and Andrew Latchford, to whom I owe a debt of gratitude, were also instrumental in publishing my book. The initial ebook was soon released in 2009, but everyone was keen to let me know that paperbacks do better than ebooks!

This writing project came about as a direct consequence of imagination, experience, broken dreams, delusions, fantasies and actual setbacks of my own. The entire writing process enabled me to get my ideas onto paper and therefore obtain some feedback from objective sources. I wrote the bulk of the script whilst living alone in a Scarborough Rethink supported accommodation flat on Sussex Street. I had been in hospital and gradually phased into independent living once again over a two year period. My personal space was perfect for uninterrupted, intellectual endeavour. I felt to be living as though human rather than spending my life under the cover of diagnosis alone. Paul Kirven offered regular email contact with Chipmunka and always kept me up to date with the proceedings. I believe he is also a Mental Health Support Worker, so Plan 103f begins there! The next chapter details my first experiences of being diagnosed with schizophrenia, as also does chapter eight.

Numerous people are responsible for helping me out along the way. To say 'thankyou' to some would be only right. David Goodwin from Terrington has been helping out since I acted in 'A Midsummer Night's Dream' 1998 in Helmsley. He went through thick and thin with professional acting and family life, and always found time to help me out. At the Ellis Centre in Scarborough, I would like to offer my gratitude to Matthew Havenhand, who helped me understand life from a grown-up angle, frequently putting a perspective on my problems where life seemed unfair or otherwise demeaning. Currently in Scarborough, my friend and musical mentor David Ives inspired me to stick to my guns on the piano where otherwise I may have simply forgotten. The staff at Rethink who helped me out whilst living in the supported accommodation flat are forever in my thoughts, for keeping my dreams alive and keeping me on track and in check. To Alex Boorman, a definite thanks, for being my mentor-friend since September 2008, reading my scripts, and attending my gigs, and Simon Muir, who helped me move on from hospital in 2007. Plus all the folk who spared a kind word, a smile, or some practical advice – these people are eternally appreciated. As are Dr Sen and Dr Mogyorosy who enabled my life to take a new course in 2007.

Blind ambition was knowing what I wanted, but not knowing how to get it, or whom to approach. The above people plus more provided a necessary bounce back for my ideas to feel real once again. Once, in an internet survey, one question asked whether I was looking for a more 'real' or a more 'famous' experience with my life. I thought about it at the time and elected for 'real'. It seems that this same question remained with me over the years, remembering in the night and wondering during the day – what of those who elected for 'famous'?

Chapter Four
Sectioned

I was sectioned, under the Mental Health Act, three times in my twenties. It all began in August 1998, at the age of 20, when my parents took me to see Dr Bridge (a consultant psychiatrist) at 'The Retreat' - a clinic in York city centre. My thoughts at the time were that I wanted to become a black belt in Taekwondo with Olympic potential, be a musical superstar, attend the Paris Conservatoire, and to study Politics, Philosophy, and Economics (PPE) at the University of Oxford, in order to go on to become Prime Minister. He told me that I had a powerful smile on my face and that he needed to speak with my parents.

The outcome of their conversation had Dr Bridge prescribing me some little orange Depixol tablets with the instruction to take one, three times a day. This, he had said, I didn't have to do if I didn't want. My parents were adamant that my serotonin levels in my brain were running too high and needed controlling with medical help. I had a chemical 'imbalance'.

Earlier that year I had lost two part time jobs, one washing dishes in a local pub, 'The Star Inn', Harome (there had been an incident with one of the waitresses), and the other working at a local garage forecourt, serving petrol and other goods to customers. The Manager had sacked me for behaving strangely in the garage. My co-worker, Mike, asked after me for years as he recognised my mum when she bought petrol.

The next four months I was in receipt of Income Support and was getting about £80 a week. At this point in time there was a lot of talk of 'The Millennium Bug', ie would it affect people going into the new Millennium? Maybe I was susceptible or something. In the event of the New Year I shut myself in my room listening to all the fireworks going off in the village. I had no interest to be there to celebrate. My emotions had failed me. Mum came upstairs to wish me a Happy New Year after midnight and I don't remember responding. We made up for that

New Year fiasco in 2010 when Mum and I attended an Open Air concert in Scarborough, featuring Jose Carreras, Dame Kiri te Kanawa, and the Opera North Orchestra, with Brian Blessed as compere. The firework finale was amazing and made up for 2000!

Anyway, within three weeks, I had shaved off all my body hair and pronounced myself to be a Millennium Baby. That was the last straw. The ambulance came to take me to hospital in January 2000. There was a police officer who wrestled me into handcuffs in my bedroom. There were three doctors and two ambulance staff. I had been lying there counting my pennies when my eldest brother Chris gave me five minutes warning.

He accompanied me in the ambulance to St Mary's hospital, Dean Road, Scarborough where I was stretchered to the solitary room, and he left me shortly after with all the doctors and nurses. I was scared and nervous. My first act was to strip off all my clothes and lie on my back on the blue mattress in the room. A doctor asked me if I knew where I was and I guessed 'Scarborough' because I knew the place from when my other brother Jonny had been there some years earlier. I then asked what was I supposed to have wrong with me and he told me 'schiz – schizophrenia'. That did it. That was the first time in my whole life that I had encountered the diagnosis, that day.

I was left on my own for a while whilst the staff talked outside the solitary room. I freaked out and blockaded the mattress against the door, screamed, shouted, and jumped up to rip the strip light from the ceiling. This caused my hand to bleed, and I wiped the blood all over my naked body.

The nurses burst back into the room to assess the damage and to restrain me on the ground. One nurse injected me with Acuphase and they stayed on top of me until I had calmed down. I only remember somebody's red shoes to this day because of that. They were distinctive amongst the crowd.

The Green Dragon

As I was knocked out by the drug they carried me to another room where I apparently slept for three days and nights straight through. All I know is waking up to an offer of croquet potatoes and a glass of water. I requested sparkling water, and somebody actually went to the shops to get some for me.

So there I was; under a Section 3 in the hospital where I would stay until July 2000. Who would I meet, what would unfold, and how would I react to the whole procedure? A traumatic time on occasion, and at others it was TV, radio, cigarettes and flirting with the girls. The ward was mixed-sex, so only the dormitories and sleeping arrangements divided the patients.

Ten years on, whilst writing this episode, my memories are still fairly vivid. I did apply to read my Hospital notes to get more specific details, but I felt upset by them and would like to say three specific things about certain CPNs, nurses, social services and especially Mental Health 'nurse authors' who presented lies, allegations, overblown exaggerations and other gross distortions of my truths.

Firstly is the fact that this, 'The Green Dragon', is my story told by myself, not the medics. Secondly is the point that in my experience the 'staff' in hospital spent too much time looking at the finger, and never at the direction in which it was pointing, ie looking to the future and moving forwards in time unto heavenly glory – they would only take the finger at face value and refuse to acknowledge my direction. And thirdly, because I enjoy musical artistry, it has to be said that 'you can take the artist away from the art, but you can never take the art away from the artist'. They had in fact removed me from the musical facilities that had accompanied much of my life up until then. Bastards!

In fact there are some whom I would never choose to set eye upon ever again, even to the extent of wishing them gone. After ten year's reflection I can honestly say that one CPN in particular, passed herself off as a CPN, but in actual fact was nothing more than a conniving conspirator. She personally stole the best years of my life (my entire twenties) – being personally responsible for every Sectioning I had. When employed it was she who fabricated allegations to have me locked away – which were not true anyway. She was neither present at the time nor was she willing to listen to me. Years later, when I had become marathon fit it was she who came to the door claiming to be a 'number one fan' but actually was there to rescind my rights and privileges and Section me. I was up for the Great North Run 2006, Amsterdam Marathon 2006, London Triathlon 2006, and potentially London Marathon 2007 at the time, and a five month Trekforce expedition in South America was scheduled for 2007 after University. All the above were denied, then when she eventually got me into hospital, all drugged up, she knocked on my door to tell me she was going to Fiji for a holiday, and guess what – we've never met since. She was an absolute piss-taker and should pay the penalty. She lied, stole and killed my dreams. I would be happy to learn of her demise.

Back to my in-patient experiences in St Mary's, there was Hugh – dancing like an Egyptian; there was John – laughing for hours at anything, telling us all about the time he scored nine goals in one football match; there was Matt – making use of his mobile phone; there was Bill – selfishly arguing over a TV magazine, then buying me a kebab to make up for it a day later; there was a Paul McCartney – not the Beatle, but he stayed close to a girl called Kate; there was Geoff, June, Tyra (whom I called 'Tiger Tyra'), most importantly Christina (whom I am now married to), José – a Portuguese aggressor shouting at me to fight him for watching the tennis on television; Paul Schofield – something of an intellectual, Paul Hood – strange character; and many more people coming and going.

As for the staff, I remember one guitarist/singer-songwriter – whom I attacked with a belt in my hand on one occasion; one who was a titch but always seemed to have a chip on his shoulder about something or other. I learned in 2007 that he had since passed away; one ex-army nurse; a pretty student nurse; a slim and beautiful nurse; and my worst nightmare CPN who came to see me on occasion. I had previously admired her legs and requested to **** her. This caused her to set up an ongoing vendetta against me. The event never manifested, anyway. Dr R Nicholson was my Consultant Psychiatrist during this time. I never did see eye to eye with him, though; one nurse had heart problems and a family to feed; one guy shouted at me for hiding my goods in a hole in the ceiling – prize wanker. One – a fat man, recently divorced; another, an ex-rugby coach, who told me off for wearing a dressing gown without tracksuit bottoms on. Maybe my legs were that great or something?

The list could go on, but that's all I remember for now. Once I wanted to post a letter and the nurses told me not to and attempted to physically stop me. I had to make a dash for it and cross the road with my letter – a bill paid for a collection of a folder entitled 'Successful Personal Investing'. I determined to collect and read this whilst there. There were three folders to collect but I stopped after the first for some reason. Probably expenses.

The Acuphase injections prevented me from speaking properly. It made my tongue not work. Mum and Dad came to visit regularly, bringing me stuff. Music and fruit especially. At that time I had been invited to St James's Palace in London to collect my Duke of Edinburgh's Gold Award certificate which had taken me three years to earn. The bastards would not let me go to attend the ceremony, so instead, Lawrie Quinn, the local Labour MP, came to visit me at the hospital, with the award. I wore a smart shirt and tie for the event and my Dad talked to him about Esperanto. It was Dad's idea for him to visit me.

There were several photographs taken throughout the afternoon, and then Lawrie left, back to politics. That was an honour indeed, I reckoned. He made an appearance just for me. I asked what his working hours were like and he said that once he had been awake for three nights straight in order to keep up to date with work commitments.

One time I was sitting in the living room area and felt like roaring like a lion, so I did. The warden came running in and told me off. One of the female patients laughed at this, then proceeded to give me a foot massage. She also asked me to do up her bra for her that night in the dormitory. It was a bit of a fumbled job. Another female patient had me writing letters to her boyfriend for her as she could not read or write. I duly charged £1 a letter and ended up making about £15 in total for this service. My writing was not strictly word-for-word either, editing the script for comic effect.

Another time, an upstairs door had been left unlocked and I discovered this route by chance. I eventually found a way out into the town, freed from hospital. I came back after visiting a pet shop and a brief walk. Jack let me back in, wondering how I had got out. I didn't know Scarborough very well at that point so I felt a bit lost whilst outside.

I had a few good friends whilst there in St Mary's hospital, 2000. One friendship, purely platonic, was with Tyra, a blonde, 30-something, smoker. We had fun playing cluedo and ended up having a hug and a cuddle. She was released and went back home to her young boys in Malton. We met once, two years later, in Malton. We only said hello, and that was all.

Most importantly was Christina, a brunette with long, luscious, straight hair. She was a non-smoker. We had an intriguing relationship whilst in the hospital. We used to stay up late together watching TV whilst everyone else was in bed. Only, a nurse would spy on us. We remained friends. On the outside, someone proposed to her and she married him very quickly on release. He had been writing to her all the time. Her dad wished it was me, but that is a story which manifested eight years later, once our lives connected again. I didn't realise it then, but we were in fact meant for each other.

Somebody took our photograph at their wedding reception. I had completely forgotten about this photograph until one day in September 2008, Christina sent me the picture by mail whilst I was living as a bachelor in a Sussex Court flat, Scarborough. She looked stunning and gorgeous in her wedding dress. I looked happy to be with her. Something that never really

The Green Dragon

happened for us became painfully apparent. Life's cruel way of moving people onto their destiny without remorse. We were soul mates in hospital and then the big eight year divide came. Moving on and simply forgetting until – boom – I can't forget anymore. We walked on the beach at South Bay and even planned the name of our children. I'm an idiot, an imbecile, a gutless, spineless bastard. Maybe I should just have stood up and said something. We have been making up for those eight years and strongly intend to heal the hurt.

Another vivid memory is of Gary di Campo, a music therapist. He organised group sessions for musicians which I really enjoyed. However, whilst I was in the hospital he was found dead at his home with slash marks on his wrists. Nobody knows what actually happened to him. I liked Gary and was sorry to hear the news.

Asides from all this, I remember only taking part in a quiz one time, 'Who wants to be a millionaire?' I got five questions right, then crashed out. Somebody called Gareth, in an art session, requested materials so he could mould his penis. Gail, the OT of the day, declined this request. We all laughed.

The food was diverse, ranging from chili con carne and curry, to salads, soup, and pies with two veg. I bought two smart shirts (Kickers and Calvin Klein) for £15 from somebody called Bob, who was in for burglary, so maybe that was not the smartest move. He showed me a stab wound on his chest which he had acquired from a 'job'.

I spent time reading and looking through quiz questions, arranging the cards on a table top. Once I bought a packet of cigarettes (10 Mayfair) and half way into the first, the nicotine gave me such a headrush that I nearly passed out. I didn't smoke much and ended up giving the rest away.

The doctors got me onto taking lots of medication, ranging from Zyprexa-Olanzapine, through Rispiradone, Quetiapine,

Acuphase depot injections, Haloperidol, Lorazepam, Sertraline, Clopixol, and possibly Clozaril amongst others.

Round about August I was told that they were going to discharge me back into the community. Somebody called Brandon drove me to Malton to look at some sheltered accommodation to live in. It was there at 25 Station Way, Malton, that I would live for the next two years, from August 2000 until August 2002. In between times came another Mental Health Section. With Brandon we discussed the times that we had attempted public speaking at some point in our lives. He seemed unimpressed by this.

In March 2001 I was offered a full-time job at Flamingo Land Funfair and Zoo for the season. The plan was to work until September and then start at Hull University where I had been offered a place to read Management or Politics. I had chosen Management as there was a Year abroad attached if I got the grades throughout.

I worked at Flamingo Land, having changed address in town, until July 2001 when I was laid off, allegedly for 'frog-marching' an offending child to security. The truth is it had never come to this anyway and I found out that the Park's security had set the whole scenario up to have me framed. Then a day later I was arrested in town for behaving suspiciously in 'Choices' video shop in Malton. From here the police took me to Malton Police Station and gave me a thorough questioning. Dr Chawla (Psychiatrist) arrived after three hours, and with a Second Opinion Appointed Doctor I was sectioned for a second time. So, from Malton police station I was taken by ambulance to Scarborough, Cross Lane Hospital, as St Mary's had been since demolished (thank God!)

I would be here for another period of six months, between July 2001 – February 2002. Only, owing to an incident where I refused to acquiesce to an injection, the police were called – arriving in their riot gear, helmets, shields and truncheons, they pinned me to the living room floor and injected me with the medicine. A nurse offered some words of compassion as I was on the ground. It turns out she was also a chief conspirator, becoming Ward Manager later on; pretending to be a friend in order to get close, but in actual fact just wanted control and power over others. She is on my list. Moments earlier I had asked if she would like a dance, and her reply was that she would have preferred to dance. The police officers carried me to the solitary room like a log and soon I was transferred to Middlesbrough to a secure ward (Bristol ward) at St Luke's hospital, for two months. So my plans were scuppered. The flip side was that I had been offered a welcome hamper when I first moved into 25 Station Way, Malton, as a token of good wishes, and the CPN cared for her own family, although this was merely because she had control. Therefore the hamper cancels itself out automatically.

What I remember about my first time in Cross Lane was as follows. July 2001, admission, lead into solitary confinement by the staff. Ambulance crew told me to walk, but I didn't so they put me in a wheelchair.

Once inside the solitary room I panicked and ran out of the room, down the corridor and my long shorts fell down to my ankles. At the far end I remember trying to kick the doors open, but to no avail. A nurse did a judo throw on me and dropped me hard on my ass. All the team jumped on me then, on each arm and leg. And along came an injection. Not sure what though. That was a cold welcome. I yelled 'F*** off' at them, and at the ambulance driver that he was a 'circus clown'.

Then came the solitary room. Two nurses were on watch duty. In my confusion I temporarily tried to score but to no avail. I sang Simon and Garfunkel's 'Bridge over Troubled Water' one time thinking it would help me get over my own troubled waters. One day, whilst back amongst the regular 'crew', I noticed how to open the front door by pressing a button. Just as I left the building a nurse came running after me. I was still fit and ran off. My wrist band came off in the chase but I was too quick for him and got away. I first nicked down a back lane, by the golf course to the 'Rosette' pub where I drank an orange J2O, then I phoned dad at home without mentioning my predicament.

I walked into town and slept rough that night on the Westborough church steps. At 1am I phoned a friend in Thirsk called 'Lossie'. She expressed concern at the time of night. I stayed on the Westborough church steps all night, drinking tea from a late night café. I had a little bit of money on me at the time. Then at 6am I caught the first train to Leeds, then onto Bradford where my cousin Jonty lived. He received the phone call at about midday and I caught a taxi to Eccleshill where he let me in.

That night we went out for a curry in a basement curry house. Really good stuff. We caught the bus back home again and stayed up late, then I went to bed. When I was awakened at 7am it was Jonty with the words "The police are here for you, you have to get up". They had turned up with an arrest warrant in their hands.

So I was taken to Bradford police station, given a hot dog and cup of tea, then transferred to a Mental Hospital in Bradford. They kept me in for the day. At one point I climbed a lamppost in the garden and swung like a monkey from the bar. I kept charging about the ward like an athlete, playing pool and joking around. Then by about 5pm the CPN appeared with another to drive me back to Scarborough – ouch! I wanted to escape from the car on the way but sat tight. Back at Cross Lane they fed me salad and orange juice before determining what to do.

That was all the excitement for a while until I decided to run off again. A young Indian, a student nurse, came after me. Our chase ended abruptly when we came across a bicycle /car crash on the main road. A young kid was being helped into an ambulance when we got there. His bike was by the side of the road so I offered to put it in the back of the ambulance. He thought I was going to steal the bike to get away. We both walked back together to the hospital after seeing that happen, and that was that.

The Green Dragon

Another time, I caught a taxi to York and figured that I would hide out in the 'jungle' – the city-people jungle. I went for a walk about and met somebody called Duncan who had previously started a fight with me whilst working at Flamingo Land. He asked how I was doing, so I told him my predicament. He too had a predicament – his girlfriend was far gone pregnant and he wanted money. We decided to have a wager on a game of snooker. £100, best of five games in the Stonebow snooker hall. He won the match 3-2 after about one and a half hours. I was gutted, but was true to our deal. I then decided to go to The Gallery nightclub and Toffs that night where we had arranged to meet. I drank, danced, chatted and crashed out. When we were kicked out in the early hours, I was immediately arrested outside the club and taken to Fulford police station, owing to evading the Mental Health Act. Maybe Duncan shitbag had made a call? They contacted Scarborough and the next day I was returned there once again.

Suddenly, one day, I was watching TV in the living room and nurse came in to give me an injection. This was the incident in more detail. I had no intention of acquiescing to this so told him to 'F*** you, you little tosser'. He went to collect more staff. Four came back soon and I hit one in the face. They did not inject me.

I figured that was all for now. But as it happens, the room was cleared as I was sat reading a newspaper on the far settee, and I lowered the issue to witness four fully-kitted riot police running towards me. They dropped me with their shields and another injected me with some anti-psychotic drug. The staff nurse spoke to me whilst I was on the ground on my face. That was comforting.

They carried me back to the solitary room like a log, and left me alone. Days later I was transferred to Middlesbrough, St Luke's hospital. Their first act was to drop me like a stone and fill me with powerful drugs as well. I didn't really stand much of a chance. I slept for days afterwards, and had wet the mattress during this time. I got up feeling a little lost and bewildered.

During this time, Paul laughed a lot, Kenny talked of horse racing, one nurse made me want a blow job – never asked, though (she was gorgeous), and witnessed the male nurses fighting amongst themselves all the time, one nurse even made a stink about a tiny piece of paper which I had discarded on the carpet. Little things like this were all very bizarre.

I remember watching TV. Two major events happened whilst I was here. On the 11th September 2001, the Twin Towers of New York were attacked by hijacked aircraft and came crashing down, causing many to lose their lives and affecting the entire world in its devastating meaning. The TV kept repeating this surreal piece of historical terrorism all day and took over every single TV channel. I had just had my breakfast at the time. Strange to think that my eldest brother Chris had been in New York a year earlier, running the 2000 marathon (3hrs 37mins). He had visited the twin towers, as well as the Empire State building and various art galleries and museums.

The second major event was England beating Germany 5-1 at football, in the world cup I believe. I spent time playing pool, table tennis, snooker, and piano in the main hall when on leave. Walking round the grounds was interesting enough, too. There was a shop on the premises which sold sweets and things, so I called in from time to time to buy other patients' stuff whilst they had to stay on the ward. I remember going to chapel one Sunday and the chaplain Mike talking to me afterwards. He also visited the wards speaking to patients who were there. One lady gave me some flapjack which she had baked.

Mum and Dad came to visit me from time to time, and brought me things to read, eat and drink. At the time I was a big fan of Lapsang Souchong tea and plum jam on toast. Mum made homemade jam which she brought in for me.

I fancied one nurse but got nowhere. Soon they decided to discharge me back to Scarborough. I was driven in a minibus back to Cross Lane hospital where I unpacked my bags and was given a room with immediate effect. I was wearing a top which

The Green Dragon

read 'moutin lover' - somebody thought it said 'mountain lover'. It was all a big joke.

This time I got friendly with a female blonde nurse, who lent me a philosophy dictionary. We sat outside on the bench discussing things in the sunshine, but I never got closer than listening to her husky voice that day in the sun.

The wards were segregated so the only male-female interactions were in the gym or at Occupational Therapy.

My friend from Malton, Tony Smith, came to see me one time. He brought me some magazines to read. That was a refreshing visit. We had actually met at St Mary's in 2000, then lived in the same house 25 Station Way, Malton, until I worked at Flamingo Land. As it happens I was returned to the same address after my time at Cross Lane, and Tony still lived there. Also residing were John Cameron, Brian Saunders, John Harris, Russell Ingram, Alex Webb, and Chris Fischer. In June 2002 four of us decided to go on a summer holiday, so Pete (staff nurse), Tony, John and myself went to Fuerteventura, Canary Islands, for a week. The sunshine was too hot and we all got burnt on the beach or whilst sunbathing on the swimming pool patio at the villa. The only green grass on the island was either on a golf course, or on a traffic roundabout. We tried to hire out some parasols on the beach but the ticket tout was playing up and didn't speak English so we eventually got three umbrellas to share. Pete and John were our drivers for the week. John had a white Audi and had been on duty getting us to the East Midlands airport, UK, to and from Malton.

Back to Tony's hospital visit to me. During this period I read Time magazine every week, enjoyed eating salads, and got on with my own thing. There was Matt, Alex, Hugh, Shaun (who ended up jumping off the cliffs and killing himself, leaving a wife and kids behind) and that was all I could remember about that. I do recall making a piece of artwork in the style of Jackson Pollack with the Occupational Therapist. The nurse with red shoes had won some big competition so we all made a celebration banner for him when he arrived in the limousine.

What else do I remember about 2001? Not a lot in fact. There were incidents throughout but none too memorable. I recall listening to a CD entitled 'Renaissance' with Hugh Thomas. It was dance music. His brother had been offered a place at Oxford University and was going to Japan within a year. Hugh had once pretended to rugby tackle me in the corridor for no real reason. For Christmas that year my eldest brother Chris bought me a Sony Ericsson mobile phone – my first ever phone. This provided me with hours of entertainment and lasted at least four years until it wore out in 2005. I gained many contacts via this phone. Eternally grateful!

In 2002, I had been offered an extended place at Hull University so decided to take it up from September onwards. Originally I would have started in 2001, but circumstances prevented that. Around this time, I stopped seeing Christina and focused on my studies. So, until August 2008 we had completely separate lives, when we met by chance in town in Scarborough. I was just walking home, and she was with her mum and three young sons. I gave her my number and the calls started coming through a few days later. Her marriage had fallen through, and I was single, so we determined to get together again. In a nutshell, we stayed together forthwith, however we experienced our trials and tribulations which will be discussed in more detail in chapters eight and ten. Twists of fate seemed to surround the two of us, as we had the rockiest start full of aggressions and domestic tensions, and then went on to move in together, have twins together, win a significant share of the Peoples' Postcode Lottery in 2010, get married, buy a car, go to see The Lion King the musical in London's West End for our honeymoon, see Elton John live at Scarborough's Open Air Theatre (June 2011), and she remained a committed and dedicated mother to the boys. I struggled to meet her standards at times and sadly I hit her at one point and this caused social services to step in and have involvement with the family. We had to live apart for quite some time, however, which caused us to question our relationship. More on us later though!

So what happened between September 2002 and August 2008? In a nutshell, an awful lot happened to both of us. I had almost five great years including college, and a year abroad, on a Canadian exchange. I also trained for and ran a marathon in April 2006. Christina had a first marriage and three young boys. In July 2006, coinciding with the end of my degree course, I had stopped taking medication in order to run my marathon and be a blood donor. The social services determined that I was unwell again so came to Section me from my parents' house in Beadlam. I ran away and eventually ended up arrested in a Swaledale field in the Yorkshire Dales, near Keld, by two police officers. They took me to Northallerton Police station where a psychiatrist evaluated me and shortly I was again taken to St Luke's hospital, Middlesbrough, to PICU (Psychiatric Intensive Care Unit) Coulby Unit. This episode is to be detailed in chapter eight.

Chapter Five
Hull Years

In September 2002 I began student life at Hull University. For my first year there I had applied to be living in a traditional hall of residence – Thwaite Hall, near Cottingham. The second year was in a shared student house at 8 Cranbrook Avenue, and the final year in 61 Grafton Street, again a shared student house. On my first night in Thwaite Hall there was a communal meeting in the Junior Common Room (JCR), lead by the wardens David Sands and Philippa. The committee was presented to us all and the ground rules layed out for the year ahead.

Some elected to stay in the hall that night, whilst others elected to go the student nightclub on campus called Asylum. I ended up going out that night but I really ought to have stayed in as there would have been plenty of time to go out later in the year.

My room was number 32 on the ground floor, a small room consisting of single bed, wardrobe, bookcase, writing bureau and radiator. A nearby kitchenette allowed for refreshments, etc, to be prepared. In the hall there was a communal dining room in which breakfast and evening dinner were on offer every day at 8am and 7pm. There was also a library and a computer room upstairs in the hall for students to use. My next door neighbour was a genial fellow from Manchester called Ciaran Murphy. He studied sports science and played guitar and football very well. At that time he was with a lovely girlfriend called Natalie. Also in Thwaite Hall was another Mancunian called Chris Morris. Both had been to the same school previously. Chris was a funny, highly intelligent guy with a penchant for smoking. He was seeing Adele from Manchester at the time and was a big Cliff Richard fan, displaying posters and calendars in his room.

Initially I was due to participate in The Great North Run, Newcastle, October 2002, so I had to make allowance for this as I had previously trained with Pickering running club and raised £500 for Leukaemia Research in the process. As it turned out I got round the course in about 2 hours, and the bus ride involved an early 6am pickup from the Rose and Crown pub in the village of Beadlam/Nawton. At the time I had intended to go on to run the London marathon, but as it transpired over the years that event never manifested. Not for lack of want or applying, though.

During my time in Thwaite I hung out with the following students: Steven Morris (Business school and football) from Bridlington, Dave Twitchell (Business school accountant, also from Bridlington), James Halls (Business school Londoner dating a beautiful girl called Emma), Ed Beecroft (Business schooler from Scarborough) who owned a very nice car and always seemed a cut above most of us. I secretly related him to the Fonz in Happy Days. We went our separate ways, but met several times in later years. Ed went on to train in Law, and ride a 1600cc road bike, but still made time to talk to me. He recommended a Fujifilm digital camera for me in 2003 which I still use to this day.

Also on my radar were Amanda Borg (went on to become JCR President), Louise Griffiths (gorgeous blonde who lived next door to me in my final year on Grafton Street), Fiona Wicks and Caroline from the Christian society who often lead the prayer groups, Fran also a similar age to myself (she asked me to dance at the end of year ball), and Rachel from the Christian Society. Another group within the hall included Adam Fernando, Mark (nicknamed Spanner), Chris (studying Forensics), then a footballer called Jonny who often took centre stage in the hall. One of the main reasons I applied to Thwaite Hall was because of its Steinway grand piano in the drawing room. I used to enjoy playing that on occasion, as well as an upright on the dining hall balcony.

In my first year I signed up for St John Ambulance First Aid with the Links society. Part of the process was to do duty shifts in the Asylum nightclub in case of injury/accident. Also events such as Remembrance Day in the city centre were attended by Links. In my year were Gemma Hindhough, Deborah Medd (The

Lawns), Charles Ockford (Clemence Hall; once went on an evening run with me), James Pepper, Dave together with Hannah, and Matthew Cooper, who all took turns in leading the proceedings. Also Lucy and Philip Wright (who was with Helen Nicholson), Susan Riley and her boyfriend Pete, amongst others. One evening I was on training with Links and back in Thwaite hall there had been a public award bestowed upon me for drinking a funnel of ale sometime previously. I got back to much amusement that evening!

Owing to my medical diagnosis I had been allocated my very own Sony Vaio laptop computer with printer and minidisk player. This arrived within two weeks of starting. I still use this equipment today – eight years on. They decided a laptop would be more practical for the year abroad, though, for mobility. I was introduced to MSN messenger and hotmail soon, and having taken a computing course in Malton in 2002 (European Computer Driving Licence) I was ready to learn the ropes. My first essay was a humble affair, but included in the appendices are my ten best pieces of academic writing, chronologically, from my time at Hull.

Moving between Thwaite Hall and campus involved either a bus ride or a walk, often depending on the weather and physical room on the bus. The Lawns students usually crowded the bus out by the time it reached Thwaite Hall.

I also joined an international student society called AISEC. Members promoted the international community and we spent time making calls and emails and attending conferences, but it didn't work out for me, so apart from a karaoke appearance at the Old Grey Mare where I was dressed as an Austin Powers gigolo singing Spandau Ballet's 'Gold', my time with AISEC was fairly fruitless.

The first year was spent exploring various pubs and clubs including The Gardener's Arms (Cottingham Road), The Railway Junction (Cottingham village), Pozition nightclub, The Piper Club, Heaven or Hell, Asylum and the Jonny Mac bar,

The Green Dragon

dedicated to the former student John McArthey who was held hostage with Terry Waite in Iran. Newlands Avenue was also full of student-oriented shops, cafes and venues, including the piano restaurant called 'Latitude'.

The Vineyard church was for me during my time at Hull. I liked their message and the form of worship using an evangelical Christian-rock band of drums, guitars, bass, keyboard and singers. I often attended the Sunday service there and made many friends at the time.

In the city itself I was privileged to attend the Deep marine life centre with my brother Chris and cousin Jonty, and also, with Ciaran and Steve, football at the KC stadium Hull Tigers v Grimsby, cinema at the Odeon with friends, ice skating at the Arena with Links, as well as ten pin bowling and Quasar Laser.

I could have used a push bike while at Thwaite Hall, but opted to walk to lectures instead. For me, the most nerve wracking moment of that year was when mum and dad left me on the first day in the Hall, surrounded by 200 other bright young students. I didn't know what to expect but I had to visit Castle Hill hospital several times for a checkup with Dr Harkness, at Mill View Court. My then social worker was called Charles, and he came to Thwaite Hall to check on me several times as well.

I enjoyed the snooker, table tennis, and unlimited music collections going around the hall. But for me, the real gratitude goes towards those who made this experience possible in the first place. In Thwaite Hall we each had a cubby hole for our post to be delivered every day. Somebody called Peter offered to keep my hair short so gave me a grade 4 on request outside the main hall one day.

I was a bit naughty with smokes and drinks on occasion, once purchasing a crate of Kronenbourg for Christmas consumption. Dad partook of a bottle while visiting, I seem to remember. There were Thwaite balls at Christmas and end of year. I was in Thwaite Hall September 2002 – May 2003.

Jamie Kershaw

The first essay that I wrote in Thwaite Hall was for the module Management and Organisational Behaviour, due date 05/11/2002. Please find that piece of work below. The best 10 pieces form the appendices later on.

*

'Any organization needs "different" people within it in order to optimise performance and effectiveness through the unique contribution of each individual'. Discuss.

To look at this title fills one with thoughts such as how obvious it would all be in an organization if everyone thought the same way and shared all the same ideas and beliefs. However, in practice such an occurrence tends to be impractical and not the way it actually is. Throughout the discussion there will be examples of actual companies related to in order to highlight the need for different people in an organization. What are 'different' people? Simply put, we are all unique and therefore have different thoughts and ideas. First let's take a look at the advantages and drawbacks of having different people working in the same organization.

Some simplistic advantages of having different people within an organisation would be that the more perspectives there are on the same situation, the more likely it is that the most appropriate or progressive outcome will be attained. For example, if Sven Goran Eriksonn decided that David Beckham should play in defence for the England team, but the rest of the squad unanimously agreed that he should remain in midfield, their collective opinion would probably persuade their manager that David Beckham should indeed remain in midfield. This is an example of how having different perspectives on any one situation could result in that which is for the best. Another simplistic advantage of having different people within an organisation would be that the more people there are present, the more specialist skills their talents would cover. For example, in a typical office of a small business there would be present something along the lines of : manager, assistant manager, secretary, receptionist, administration, IT specialist, cleaner, and possibly a few patrons too. From this list one can identify the necessity for having different people with different skills in the same organization. Without their unique specialist skills the organization would not be able to function as a whole, fully synergised company. A further advantage is that no matter what else in life we are all unique, we are all specialists in one way or another like it or lump it. One enters the world with nothing, one leaves the world with nothing so as collective as many situations appear to be in life we are all on our own for better or for worse. But how does that answer the question? It insinuates that to begin with in a career we may feel different from the 'others' whilst in actual fact being a team player but at the same time understanding our value as a unique individual with a critical part to play in the running of the organization. We are all key players whether actually being a high-fallutin' manager or a mundane cleaner. So long as we appreciate this whilst undertaking a profession within an organization life seems *more* somehow.

"Organizations are social settings in which people interact with their colleagues. They are NOT collections of isolated individuals making decisions and taking action in splendid solitude." (Pfeffer, J. 1992) Therefore different people with different ideas are essential towards a fully functional organization. This leads onto the phrase 'interpersonal influence' because organizations clearly rely on all of their employees to produce the goods and get the job done. An organization would expect of its employees head-strong, independent and creative thought in order for the necessary progress to be made. We are all influenced by many factors in our lives eg the people close to us (such as family and friends), those we see on television, those we hear on, or about on, the radio, and those we read about in newspapers and magazines. The media influences our lives enormously. This is a solid example of interpersonal influence ie how others affect our lives and have influence on us. Following on from this one could say that the world of business organizations is a social interdependence where people succeed by factors such as co-operation, determination and motivation. 'Different' people can act as a source of motivation by leading by example, not taking 'no' for an answer, and being quite single-minded about one's own thoughts and ideas to be carried out. Motivation in this fashion could be said to optimise performance and effectiveness through each individual within the organization; all the more so because each individual provides a unique contribution to the organization and as a whole team of employees create the company's working power.

Synergy occurs as a consequence of interaction and interdependence of the people within an organization. Without synergy and employee collaboration a business would collapse. In addition to this is the communication factor, without which the business could not operate. Different people combine to make this synergy. If everyone were to be on the same wavelength the business would be at risk of falling flat and employees would lose interest in the organization. However where people merge with different 'wavelengths' (by this I mean different thoughts and ideas) and are interdependent, a synergy is formed which makes the company perform as effectively as possible. Different people communicate in alternative ways, with an understanding of which allows people to make sense of the communication made by one another. Methods of communication include : body language (physical gestures), spoken word (talking and listening), written word (reading and writing), visual images (powerpoint presentation or slide show), multimedia (IT, newspapers, TV etc).

Let's take for an example a hotel. The problems that would arise if everybody thought the same could be as follows. For example if every employee wanted to be a chef in the hotel's kitchen what would become of the waiters, bar staff, receptionist, administration, cleaners, management and so on? The answer is that the hotel would rapidly dissolve into oblivion if no-one was willing to take on these 'different' roles within the organisation.

It would not be possible for every employee to be a chef – that old saying is true "too many cooks spoil the broth" (anon).

Another example could be an Arts centre. Many people desire to be a world-class international performer in one field or another, but in reality it is not possible for everybody to do so. Consequently there is a necessity for the staff of an Art's centre to do their job effectively eg stage lighting and sound systems, administration (organises who performs where and when), Director (responsible for the organization as a whole), and any patrons who actively fund such a centre. There are of course many more roles to fill in the functioning of an active performing art's centre but this is just a brief example to highlight the necessity of 'different' people in an organization.

A third example could be a garage. What would happen if all the staff wanted to be an ace mechanic and waylaid the other jobs such as receptionist, secretary, manager, fuel-attendant and so on? The garage would not be able to operate efficiently unless it happened to be specifically a 'mechanic's garage' solely for the purpose of repairs/MOTs and has no known administration practice. The chances are that this garage would not be too popular if their clients did not know where they stood in terms of having their vehicle seen to.

These three examples show how important it is for different individuals to play their own part in the running of an organization and to give it their absolute devotion and concentration in order that the 'whole' works. Organizations need to evolve. They do this by changing, and in order that change be made there must essentially be different people working together with their own unique ideas about how a company should operate. In implementing change there are Sponsors – deciding who should carry out the change; Champions – leaders of the change programme; and Players – those who actually carry out the change. In this context the hierarchy can be seen to be necessary in order that the subordinates carry out their allocated functions properly and efficiently.

So to conclude the advantages of having 'different' people within an organization it is reasonable to say that to optimise performance and efficiency in an organization there must be 'different' people within.

Now let's take a look at the drawbacks of such a situation. Known as the 'horns and halo' effect, we prefer to say 'yes' to the requests of people we already know and like. Liking being based on the following : 1) social similarity, 2) physical attractiveness, 3) compliments and flattery, 4) contact and co-operation, 5) association with other positive things such as bringers of good news. (Cialdini) From this one could draw the conclusion that the more similar people actually are, the more agreement and nodding of heads would occur than for different people where arguments, debate, combat and conflict are more likely to occur. Also known as constructive criticism, this is in theory more likely to occur where there are real differences of opinion, progressive thought patterns may not actually occur where people are too like-minded.

Some other simplistic drawbacks of having 'same' people in an organization could be as follows…..the working environment would be exceedingly dull and sameish to be a part of ie nobody would actually want to change everything as it would all be pre-agreed upon. There would be an exceedingly limited amount of perspectives to see the issue from, where in practice it is crucial to get as many differing perspectives as possible in order that the most effective outcome is attained.

One possible risk of having 'same' people within an organization is that there may be a tendency to be too intimate in the workplace thus detracting from the significance of the work to be done in the organization. We are all only human after all but there is a line concerning employee's intimacy which should not be crossed in an organization's daily functioning. Similarly to the above point is the tendency to make jokes. Nothing wrong with having a laugh, but if it is at the expense of somebody else that could affect the working etiquette. Similar-minded people may do exactly that – make fun of one another at their own expense. It's a proven fact that laughter is good, but one should bear in mind what one is laughing about. These are some simplistic drawbacks of having 'same' people within an organization.

A drawback of having 'different' people within an organization is that certain situations are likely to result in ambiguity because the individuals concerned will have a different understanding on the situation/circumstance. Some people are born risk-takers and can therefore be the making or the breaking of a company. Were everybody to think the same way there may be less or even no risks taken, therefore no functional organization would be created in the first place. This leads me on to the example of one Mr Robert Moses of the USA. If we were all the same, the chances are that many wonders of the world would not be created, purely because people would be satisfied with their lot at the present moment thereby reducing motivation for change and improvement. Robert Moses (perhaps one of the worlds most influential men of the 20th Century) , as an enormous creative power built 12 bridges, 35 highways, 751 playgrounds, 13 golf courses, 18 swimming pools and more than 2 million acres of parkland in New York city; all during the space of a 44 year career cycle. Of course he had teams of builders to actually construct those items but the point is that he, as a different individual, decided that he was going to make a significant change and impact on everybody's lives and set about making those enormous changes. Had he been a like-minded person the projects that he set out for himself to undertake would more than likely not have been created at all. It was his creative powers and self drive that enabled such constructions to occur.

Different people arrive into the organization with different goals and different ideas, thus potentially expanding the company's dimensions as their goals are realized. However the goal must be meaningful otherwise nobody else would take it for real ie noone would take you seriously if the goal was not meaningful to others as well as to oneself. People with super-egos often have great independent creative thought processes, consequently organizations get formed and employees come running to see what all the fuss is about. An interesting question that could be considered as an essay title within itself, but can be linked to this chosen title is "Why is it that with a common culture and educational system people display different characteristics?" (Eysenck, 1982) There is of course no short answer to this question but it is in fact relevant to this essay's chosen title by looking into why people behave differently whilst coming from similar educational backgrounds.

There are four principal types of people in terms of mood, social conduct and behaviour. They are:

> *Sanguine* (optimistic and confident)
> *Phlegmatic* (practical and unemotional)
> *Melancholic* (depressive or having an eye for detail)
> *Choleric* (hot-headed or angry in character)

From this short list we are able to better define why certain people behave in a different way from others. In addition to which is the ratio between extrovert and introvert. At one end of the scale an extrovert is likely to be out-spoken and relatively noisily sociable to be around, whereas at the other end of the scale an introvert would seem reserved and quietly timid to be around. But we are what we are and to a certain extent we have the capability to change ourselves just so long as it doesn't adversely affect others. We live in a social world after all and people are always on the look out for communication such as gossip and scandals which could be brought to the forefront of ones attention. So different people look out for other people's news and what they may be striving towards in the future. This often grabs our attention whether in the headlines of a newspaper or spoken word by a busy-body next-door neighbour.

Let's take for example a commercial garden and look at why there would be drawbacks to have different people working there. In a garden there is very much work to be done 24 hours a day, 7 days a week. What if someone amongst the staff were to decide 'I'm different therefore I should be exempt from pulling up weeds and keeping a track on which crop is growing where'.

An instant result would not make too much difference, but within a relatively short period of time the garden would start to get messy and tangled and other gardeners would look upon the guy who has assumed his own importance in being different from the others. It is more than likely that before long this gardener's place at the commercial garden would be under threat of losing his job by reason of not being actively involved enough with the practical aspect of the job. So in a garden they need like-minded people who are willing to get their heads down and get the job done.

So to conclude the drawbacks to having 'different' people in an organization it could be said that too many perspectives cause ambiguity and rational decisions are harder to make.

In conclusion to the essay as a whole I agree with the title that an organization does indeed need different people to optimise performance and effectiveness.

(word count: 2598)

References

Alexis/Wilson (1967) *Organizational decision making* - Prentice/Hall
Cronje/Du Toit/Motalta (2000) *Introduction to business management*
Donaldson L (2001) *The contingency theory of organizations*
Gilgeous V (1997) *Operations and the management of change*
Heller R/Hindle T (1998) *Essential manager's manual*
Lessem R (1988) *Intrapreneurship*
March J G (1988) *Decisions and organizations* - Blackwell
Martin J (2001) *Organizational behaviour* - Thomson learning
Murphy M (1996) *Small business management*
Pettigrew A/Fenton E (2000) *The innovating organization*
Pfeffer J (1992) *Managing with power* - HBS
Rahim M A/Golembiewski R T/Pate L E (1997) *Current topics in management*
Torrington D/Hall L/Taylor S (2002) *Human resource management*

*

During the interim summer holiday, June/July 2003 I attended a cathedral camp in Gloucester where a group of young volunteers joined forces for a week to renovate parts of Gloucester cathedral. We slept in dorms and shared the catering duty between us each night, with two chefs on a rota every day and a dinner budget of £30-£35 all in. I had been meaning to do a cathedral camp since 1997 so was happy to finally have the opportunity to be there.

At the end of the week I caught the train to London and stayed in Chiswick with my eldest brother Chris for some time, attempting to find work but ending up helping him serve wine at summer concerts and prepare homes for refurbishment as he was a professional carpenter. Mum visited at one point as we had tickets to see some live Wimbledon tennis during that summer!

The Green Dragon

From September 2003 – June 2004, back in Hull, I lived at 8 Cranbrook Avenue with Lee Johnson (he was born with a gammy leg so walking was a challenge), Ryan Britten (diagnosed with leukaemia, good at darts and driving his Lexus car), Jenny (a medic who had a brief liaison with Ryan), and Alison (drama student). On occasion we all went out to the cinema or supermarket, eg Tesco or Asda. Transport was either by bus or Ryan's car. One film was a legal thriller starring Gene Hackman which we couldn't make much sense of.

This year really counted for me as I needed to get the grades to qualify for the following year abroad. I got a routine going of gym, tennis and badminton clubs, AU nights out, meditation, and reading as much as possible. With the Athletic Union (AU) we went on social nights to pubs and clubs in the city, some of which offered discounts for students.

I remember Rishi (Tennis President 2003/04) and Amy (Badminton President 2003/04), Andy Riley (nicknamed Nur), Andy Campbell, Ade Webb (dancer and folk guitarist extraordinaire), Vicki, Leila, Shona Lloyd (went onto become Student President 2005/06), Suzanne Riley and boyfriend Pete, Paul, and James Grudgings (just back from an exchange year to Australia). He sold me a new grip for my tennis racket.

During the year I loaded my entire CD collection onto my laptop. This took weeks to do in preparation for some portable home entertainment abroad the next year. One time I prepared a hot curry for all the household, charging £3/head. There were no complaints and lots of empty plates afterwards.

Family members made visits at various times during the year. I kept my bike in the garden shed as my main mode of transport, often getting to and from the gym. My brother Jonny stayed over one weekend with his friend Alan. Another time, my brother Chris came up from London and stayed over along with cousin Jonty for a couple of nights. Dad called in once and offered to sell a saxophone to Ryan. I made friends with an author/student called Chaz Blackburn who had written a book entitled 'Trouble', in which he talked of his experiences living in London.

Shona hosted some house parties during this year and I went along to several, enjoying the music, food, drink and company. She lived with a guy called Richard Collingsworth (cricket/tennis). He once paraded round the city nightclubs dressed as a tiger! From one house party I had somehow managed to end up at Napoleon's casino along with three others. I had a modest flutter on the roulette but nothing came from that. We often attended the Asylum nightclub on campus with the other students. We attended comedy nights and fancy dress parties on occasion. One time I posed as the Gatekeeper, but ended up disowned in the Pozition nightclub so had to make my own way home that night. Another time I wore a bright red Hawaiian shirt as it was supposedly a Hawaiian night, but only a few of us dressed for it. These nights out made up for having no TV to watch.

I was still with Links First Aid that year and briefly had a post as Training Coordinator, but that fell through shortly owing to others wanting it more than myself. I did several duty shifts in the Asylum nightclub during the year. On a Links social Christmas party I dressed up as Robin from Batman. Costumes were available from Tony at the 'Dressing Up Box'.

My Personal Supervisor was Graeme Reid (also disability tutor). He helped enormously with preparations and advice for coursework, etc. Other lecturers from this year whom I can still remember were David Tucker (Business School Director), Gabrielle Vosseberg (organised all exchange years), Giovanni Andresani, Tony Bosco, Dr Peter Murray, Mandy Brown, Marianne Afanassieva, Deborah Johnson, John Nicholson, Christopher J Hammond, et al. Many staff taught us throughout the course of the three years at Hull.

I had applied for an exchange year, so was instructed to choose five possibilities from which one would occur. I chose Australia, Canada, and three in the USA. I was put forwards for an exchange year at Dalhousie University, Halifax, Nova Scotia, Canada. This is the subject matter for chapter six (following this). I had acquired the necessary qualifications from the second year!

However, following my return to the UK I had one final year remaining at Hull. For this I contacted the Accommodation Warehouse and they gave me a room at 61 Grafton Street, along with Andreas (a German engineering student who beat me at snooker), Norah Garvie from Sierra Leone, and three Chinese students Ji, Alan and his girlfriend Stacy. Another self-catering year lay ahead.

My two extracurricular goals for this final year were to run a marathon and to attend the world-famous Anthony Robbins firewalk seminar in London. I had applied for the London marathon but got turned down again, so took up brother Chris's suggestion and applied for the Paris marathon instead. They offered me a charity place for Get Kids Going, April 2006. On condition of raising £895 I was in. So I did! This feat forms the basis for chapter seven in this book.

Some nights I went out with Norah to sing karaoke. I was still hanging onto my overseas relationship with Taya Krivoruchko from the exchange year, though, so could only suffer. I attempted Marvin Gaye's 'Ain't no mountain high enough', Paul McArtney's 'Live and let die', and the tribute song to John Peel 'Teenage kicks'. They all went badly, so I felt like a muppet.

At one point I was digging in the garden and found an old bone and some broken porcelain, so cleaned them up and took them to the local artefact museum for analysis. I thought that they might be of interest, but the bone was just from an old Sunday roast.

Back on track, in order to acquire and maintain fitness for the marathon, I frequently got up early in the morning to go to the gym, play squash, run in Pearson Park, or swim. I regularly used meditation, yoga, deep-breathing, tai chi, leg massage, and took careful note of my diet in detail. On Monday evenings I went to the sports hall for circuit training. It was early one morning in Pearson Park that I met a group of students who told me their housemate Ben Dudgeon was training to run the London marathon at the same time. Ben was a drama student.

They all shared a big house in Pearson Park. I also met Oliver Ramos from Portugal, living there. He sponsored my cause very generously with £30! We got on well for several months then he returned to Portugal, and I have never heard from him since. I once clambered over some railings to get to the park but somebody had painted fresh black paint on so my hands and t-shirt got covered. After the marathon I went to see Ben and Olly. Ben was driving a Mini Cooper, Olly riding a pushbike; both had spare for me, so what do I choose?....the spare bike of course – I couldn't stop training for some reason!

I joined the Athletics Club 2005/06, Presided over by Richard Vickers (who also attended the Vineyard church on occasion). We sometimes trained at the Costello Stadium as a group. We took part in races ranging from the 10km in Broughton, to the Bridlington Half-marathon. I completed that course in 1hr 46mins (November 2005). Once I walked to Beverley (and back), 10km each way, for their annual road race. I watched that year, 2006, and participated the next, 2007, after time out. Another time I cycled to the Westwood pastures in Beverley where the athletics club were training. I ran with them barefoot in the muddy grass for the session before cycling back to Hull once again. Everyone else was in cars so I had double fitness at the time. I used my pushbike a lot, and rollerblades, although security had a problem with me using them on campus. I played squash early on a morning and often won my games. Following the marathon I was appointed President of the Athletics Club. Again, a short-lived honour which lasted about 3 weeks, as I was approaching another unforeseen breakdown in my life.

That year I had a big problem. That problem was Harry Barkas (Norah's Greek love affair). Either he didn't like me from the outset, or he had figured I was trying for Norah. We were merely housemates. Either way, one evening his friend Harris had stolen a squash ball from my collection so I asked for it back. From this a whole series of events unfolded. In a nutshell, for whatever reason, he came at me several times with fists flying – maybe I did the same back – I got a bloody lip from the first incident. Then as I was due to leave for Paris he left a note on my door asking me to clean the bathroom. I had to go, so I left. When I came back after the weekend away he had burst my bike tyres so I went up to query this. He came down in greko boxing gear and proceeded to go at me hard in the living room. I was dazed for a while but could move on still. Alan heard the fuss and came downstairs to break it up and see what was going on.

Some time passed and I had been willing to let bygones be bygones, but the third, final and most disturbing occasion came some weeks later. I was in the kitchen having a meeting with HUAC when Barkas gatecrashed. He yelled a list of allegations followed by a statement for me to be home tonight. Then he left with Harris, our HUAC meeting closed instantly and I was alone again. We had been applying for the next year's club budget at the time.

To keep it brief, he did come back with Harris that evening. I was in my room, he kicked the partially open door wide open and proceeded to hit me hard in the head on my bed, then threw the full sponsorship containers at my head, then tried to drag me by the ankles. He challenged me to go to the living room where something was in store for me. I locked my door and scarpered through the window onto the streets of Hull where some passersby took concern over my bloodsoaked face/t-shirt and called an ambulance. I was driven to Anlaby Road Hospital for a checkup but didn't want to be there so walked home again late at night and cleaned myself up.

That was it; my head was all over the place from then on. I couldn't focus or concentrate on my final exams anymore. Steve Braund's Strategic Management went out the window…literally!

Social Services and my parents kept showing up at the door to check up on me, and wanted to take me to Castle Hill Hospital for a psychiatrist to evaluate me. I wasn't letting this happen all over again. Consequently I put on a brave face and persisted in sending them away, before finally the housing contract expired and I had to go home.

To be fair, I had gone a bit nuts, in an attempt to step my life up a gear to something more significant – to make history – I was cracked up burning old bank statements and baking assorted produce, then offering it round with some kind of Christian allusions. Maybe the whole Barkas fracas was him trying to crucify me owing to my then religious leanings. Either way, whatever it all was about, it put the shits up me.

At one point the next door neighbours had a party to which I was invited. In fact I was getting paranoid about mingling with others, so stayed home. Andy, (nicknamed Mowgli), whose party it was, played hockey and was also in Thwaite Hall when I was there three years earlier. Louise Griffith also lived next door by now. I regularly attended 'cell groups' with the Vineyard church crew. I admired John, Fiona, and Caroline in particular for their convictions in faith. Some evenings we would distribute goods on the street to advertise the church. The pastor Jeremy had previously been a big name in the music industry, being a key agent in signing the 80s rock legends Queen.

In Grafton street I was learning guitar, harmonica and electric portable keyboard. This flipped my housemates out though, sometimes playing and singing in the bath as well. The 90's band The Beautiful South originated from Hull's Grafton Street! After my beating I once blockaded myself in the house by barraging the fridge-freezers and drying machine against the front door. Ji complained about this. I was getting really paranoid and sticking around a darkened room a lot. One time on a walkabout, I was cutting through Pearson Park and I witnessed a racist fight where a drunk and angry white man smashed a glass beer bottle on a black man's head. I contacted the local constabulary who proceeded to do a full identity check on me, taking over half an hour to arrive at the scene by which point the brawl had ended with a crowd pinning the white man down in an alleyway. I was unnerved by this.

Rather than catch a bus to town I spent the entire year on foot, preferring to walk the 3 miles to town every time. At Sainsburys for breakfast in the early hours one morning I was told to hurry along by the security staff, so gave them an earful about the bullshit policies of Sainsbury's. He then escorted me to the door, having leapt over the counter first.

Owing to being on a sponsorship spree for the charity concerned (Get Kids Going), I took a liberal view on who might sponsor me and what they would sponsor me. I applied for and received sponsorships ranging from money, clothes, fruit basket, chest hair removal, free drinks/snacks, to people sending me downloaded music on the internet. I also got rejections and was once threatened with a flying chair in the Zoo café on Newlands Avenue. The proprietor thought I was a nutcase and called the police, but I went before they arrived.

I gave some charity containers to several local health food shops, the student gym, the Costello stadium and the student union shop. There were hundreds of pounds raised like this. Andy owned a shop called The Good Life, and fully supported the cause, which was great because I often bought food from there at the time.

In my final year, lectures seemed less overbearing and I was able to contribute from time to time in class. I took an Independent module, learning Spanish from scratch at beginner's level. Groupwork enabled students to bounce ideas off each other. A French girl called Nadila gave me a CD of Damien Rice's 'O' album. I quite fancied the lovely blonde Rhiay but she thought I was nuts so we merely worked together in the group. During that year I went to York City library and borrowed a book entitled 'The Road Less Travelled' by Dr Scott M Peck. I read this avidly, and also hired some piano music with the idea that one day I should like to sit a piano diploma. During my final year I was involved in the Procter and Gamble Universities

Business Challenge. The Hull team reached the semi-finals but I was out of my depth when we got to Newcastle for the contest.

This is a summary of my time at Hull University, but you probably get the picture. For details of my top ten pieces of university work, please refer to appendices. I shall now write of my year in Canada.

Chapter Six
Dalhousie

Based on my student experiences whilst living at Apartments 3207 & 3310, 5599 Fenwick Street, Halifax, Nova Scotia, Canada.

Semester One: September 2004 – December 2004

My farewell party was spent in London on Saturday 4th September 2004 at my eldest brother Chris's place. He cooked me a steak and chips dinner, washed down with some full-bodied red wine (probably Merlot). So, into the unknown…..would I ever return? As it transpired, I would be, even though the London bombings of July 2005 were less than a fortnight before that.

As Chris dropped me off at the local underground tube station the next morning, we bade each other adieu (in a similar fashion to the rest of the family back home in Yorkshire) with a bear hug, a back slap, and a "Look after yourself – take care!"

Once I reached Heathrow, the whole process was smooth-running, and I boarded my plane, on Sunday, September 5th , flying via St John's Newfoundland to Halifax, Nova Scotia where Dalhousie University had offered me one year as an exchange student to read a Business Management degree. An exciting revelation from my previous existence. Some students were really envious of me, I can vouch for that.

The flight lasted approximately 9 hours in total, including the changeover, with *'Shrek 2'* as the in-flight movie. We took off from Heathrow airport at 12:30pm and finally landed in Halifax, Nova Scotia at 17:30 pm Canada time. On board I met fellow students from Iran, Sweden, and Nigeria, all heading to Dalhousie University. I met my first exchange-year friend Hamoon on this flight.

At the airport our arranged contacts didn't turn up to give us a lift, so the four of us shared a taxi cab taking the one hour journey into town to the Fenwick apartments, where our year's accommodation lay ahead.

We were signed-in, registered, given the keys, and then it was up the express elevator to the 32nd floor where the 'Internationals' were due to reside. I was located in room 3207, that is, room 07 on the 32nd floor. Here I met Matt and Amy (also from Hull University on exchange).

The first night a group of us students took a general walk-about of campus and town and we ended up at Pogue Fado's, an Irish Bar. There, our group included Swedish, German, Australian, Norwegian, Chinese, English, Canadian, Danish, and Malaysian students. So, truly a cosmopolitan bunch. There I first sampled Canadian Beer, of which the choices proved innumerable – Rickards, Molsons, Labatts, Coors, Keiths, Sleemans and other cool ones, too. Very refreshing!

Having been up early back in the U.K. to catch the flight in the first place, flown over, and then spent the night out on a four hour time difference, I reckon that I had been going a full 24 hours on this day by this point. So I walked back with the other students and went to bed, feeling exhausted, at 2.30am.

The first week at Dalhousie was all about orientation and finding ones feet. On the International floors that Semester were Kate and Amanda from Australia, Hamoon and Govind (two Malaysian boys), Elizabeth, Mahim and Richard from Sweden, Per Johannes also from Sweden, Chris and Andy from Keele University, UK, Lars, Lotte and Jesper from Denmark, Carina from Germany, Yvonne and Christine from Malta, Matt, Amy and myself from Hull University, U.K., Hans from Germany, Sophie and Charles from Bath University, U.K., Naneke on a work placement from Holland, and Linus and Nikolai from Sweden, too. The floors beneath numbers 33 and 32 contained many Canadians and Americans.

A very interesting prospect to find myself in such circumstances, I thought. Much of my time was spent in the company of two American girls, Jennifer and Annie, from Texas, studying Law, and the two boys from Malaysia, who were reputed to be gay, studying Social Sciences; also, Leah and Kirsten, two girls from Germany, and a friend whom I met at the introductory orientation events. During this event there was a talent night where students were expected to get up and give some form of entertainment on 'being passed the baton'. When my turn came I attempted Tom Jones's *"What's new pussycat"*. It went down surprisingly well, even though I am no Welshman!

September was very exciting with Ice Hockey matches (Canada's National sport) to attend between the Halifax Mooseheads and the Prince Edward Island Rockets, or the Cape Breton Screaming Eagles. Tickets cost between $9.50 and $13.50 depending on the seating. During the half-time interval there would be commercial vehicles driving on the ice to advertise their brand of car, so that, plus all the overhead noise kept everyone entertained for a full 20 minutes before play resumed. We also had the privilege of watching the world championship final between Canada and Finland on a giant cine screen in our living room lounge area. Canada won – happily! Also, with this cine screen as a chief focal point, we would frequently watch movies together as well on an evening. Films such as Dodgeball, Lemony Snickett's tale of misadventures, Iris, The Big Blue, Starsky and Hutch, Hotel Rwanda, or 28 Days Later, to name but a few.

My 26th birthday on September 27th was celebrated in the company of a group of students at *"Hoagie's Steak House"* on Quinpool Road, where I made a short, but informed, speech wishing everybody well with a "new environment, new friends, new experiences, and a whole new world to explore". We all made a point of clubbing together for people's birthdays during semester, so there were also parties for Naneke, Annie, Per Johannes, Linus, Amy, and numerous others whom I haven't recorded.

By now I was fast friends with the Americans especially. One of our first nights out together was to the Khyber club, where a live band provided the entertainment. We also went to the cinema together and watched The Incredibles, and Ray (a biography of the musical legend Ray Charles). Later in the year at the cinema I saw Alexander, the historical drama of Alexander the Great, and Hitchhiker's Guide to the Galaxy, the night before Mario flew back home to Mexico. Also, Opa's, the Greek restaurant, saw a visit from our group once.

My Semester One modules which I had registered for with Timothy Richards (co-ordinator) were as follows: Marketing Communications (Professor Bob Fisher), Business in a Global Context (Jason Pendlebury, who was simultaneously teaching the module and studying for a Master's degree. He was dead keen that everybody 'cite your sources using APA referencing format'), Organizational Change, and Database Design (for which the names of the professors escape me). The first two listed modules I found absolutely fascinating, with presentations, televised/videoed advertisement-commercial making, and constructive contributions thoroughly supported, in general, as well. The third and fourth of these modules were rather more tedious so I felt less motivated to do well. The Marketing Professor had a real sense of humour and direction, which was a bonus. He provided an interesting format with clearly-expected criteria. Two memorable marketing projects were on Rolling Stone magazine, and Air Miles. The Killam Memorial library struck me as being particularly impressive with its spacious meeting area and enormous million-book collection. One room was devoted entirely to Canadian newpapers and quiet reading. I enjoyed my time reading here with a coffee. As a money-saver I shared the cost of my books with Lotte as we both read the same modules that semester.

A September trip that we made as a 'Fenwick' group was to go out on a boat around Halifax harbour – the deepest natural harbour in the world. Boats and ships such as the QE2 call in from time to time amidst their Atlantic jaunts. Also, locally a *'Harbour Hopper'* can drive you around town and then turn into a boat and pilot you around the harbour on the water! We went on a fishing boat where they checked the lobster nets out in the bay, as Nova Scotia lobster is world famous. We had intended to 'Whale-watch' but no whales surfaced this time.

The very first excursion in orientation week was to be to Peggy's Cove where we found a famous lighthouse located on LOTS of large rocks. Reputedly on occasion if you look hard enough you can see whales rising out of the water or thrashing their tails about. On this occasion there were none, so we made do with a beautiful North Atlantic panorama instead, -blue skies, sunshine and a cold, bracing wind. I bought my first postcard and sent it home to Mum and Dad from Peggy's Cove. Here I met Charles 'Chaz' from New Zealand. Hans showed an interest in visiting another local coastal settlement called Lunenburg, as the original inhabitants all came from his native land, Germany.

Interestingly, all the way from the U.K., I already had a contact in Canada. Ruth Bowman and her then boyfriend Paul Connell were in the process of building a barn to live in, with horses, dogs and a whole lot of land to keep as well. At the time the two of them were living in a tiny cold cabin and working their socks off to get this place built as much as possible before the freezing winter came. I helped them with some fence-making and cement-laying a couple of times. Jill and David, Ruth's parents, flew across to visit in October/November. We all met up for something to eat in a local café and toured the University Campus as well. This time was very special for me. I remember talking to David about Nova Scotia lobster and Symphony Nova Scotia, the regional orchestra. We looked in the campus art gallery and enjoyed a cultural time together. David had spent most of his life working at, or with, music - conducting, playing, writing, teaching, designing and creating amazing things. He was Music Director at Ampleforth College for at least twenty years, made architectural designs for the Music School, wrote many bestselling music books and raised his family with Jill. Jill taught music and Directed the Music School at York Minster Choir School for many years. Together they enjoyed a supreme style of living. Jonan, their son (my age) now lives in New Zealand and has a son, Felix, close to his heart. Ruth still lives in Canada, though is with a new partner. She works full time with horses, stables and hosts Olympic Dreams!

The view from the top of the Fenwick tower apartment block was four-fold. On one side you could see the harbour, and often at night the ships' horns would sound in the fog; on the far side you could see the Citadel of Halifax and the city lights when dark outside, and from another side the McKenzie Bridge (one of two suspension bridges crossing the harbour with a toll to pay) named after a previous Canadian Prime Minister. When I was there Paul Martin was in office, living in Ottawa, the political capital of the country. Also on the other side, the view looked directly onto the general hospital with an enormous banner on the wall advertising and promoting healthy living for all.

October saw two big parties on the international floors of Fenwick: a *lobster party* and a *fancy-dress party*. To begin with the lobster party…we counted all in and headed off to Sobeys, the local superstore, and Atlantic superstore to compare prices. Both markets sell live lobsters in the fishmonger's section of the store, stored in tanks. With Hans and PJ we bought several lobsters for ourselves then returned to tell the others from where and for how much they could buy their lobsters. This acquisition process took maybe two hours as people were very choosy about their lobster! All in and back to the floor.

How best to give lobsters their last hour? We decided that the best thing was to put them on the floor and allow them to race or at least walk freely for 15 minutes before the cooking began. As it happens, none of the lobster were really in the mood for moving too much, as though they just knew something terrible was about to happen to them. Anyhow, one by one they went in the pot and we all ate lobster with fresh baked baguettes and white wine. Nobody actually cried, but some people seemed a bit upset by the lobsters' fate.

The end of the month, Saturday 30th October, saw a remarkable fancy-dress party on the floor. We had pirates (Richard and

Andy), cowboys (Jesper), cowgirls (Katie and Amy), Charlie's Angels (Elizabeth and Mahim), celestial angels (Yvonne and Christine), glo girl with fluorescent pink hair (Annie), cat in the hat (me), a clown (Lotte), Caesar (Charles), the little devil (Amanda), Luggage labelling (Jennifer), Royal Navy seaman (Ulrich), a surgeon (PJ), a vampire/Dracula (Lars), gay drag queens (couple of French guys), gothic dress and many other original presentations. I remember talking with another Jamie from Canada about Esperanto (the topic for my Marketing project). He seemed genuinely interested. Cynical though, but an educated mind with an interested ear for things of political significance. He was dressed like Arnold Scwarzenegger that night...suave jacket with matching trousers, and a barrel chest to promote the clothing.

Throughout the semester Chris from Keele and Kate from Australia coupled together, spending many a happy moment with everyone. She had her own special birthday celebration that semester inbetween thespian drama studies. Everyone came to it to celebrate with her. I learned that they later split up when Chris flew to Australia. Kate left him then, of all times. Women!?

Elizabeth and Mahim were like sisters together, with Richard protecting them both. Linus invited his brother from Sweden to the party, and they were the only two not in fancy dress. Nobody complained about that, though. Jennifer and Annie, both from Texas, were also like sisters. Jennifer comely and Annie a slender Asian. Nanneke was here on a work experience placement with a local Occupational Therapy department in a hospital. She seemed to fit in perfectly well with everybody, anyway.

The final 'shindig' on Saturday, 16th October, was to go white water rafting on the Shubenacadie river. The river has a daily tidal bore which sweeps up the river and causes great waves to flow upstream. The Canadians cottoned onto this fact and began taking out boat trips in boats with an outboard motor. The tri[s were popular with students and adrenaline junkies alike, and we drove there one wet, rainy morning along the highway for 2 hours in 3 separate cars packed with crazy students.

Once we arrived we were kitted up with floatable wetsuits, bright orange in colour, and stripped down to shorts and t-shirts underneath. Then we walked to the boat house and clambered into our respective 'flotacles'. The entire afternoon was spent on the river getting exceedingly wet but, surprisingly, not too cold (at the time). Once the bore had passed us upstream we all jumped into the river to test our flotation suits…they worked well!

Back on dry land we trudged to the living area where we were blessed with a hot shower, dry, warm clothes, and a barbecued lunch, with hot cocoa to sip by the round log fire. We all sat around for an hour talking and cracking jokes amongst ourselves before returning to Halifax, content in our ways.

Thanksgiving in North America is an enormous affair. As I spent much time hanging round with the American girls, we (myself, Jennifer, Annie, Hamoon, and Govind) headed to a posh restaurant to celebrate the event together on Monday 11th October on returning from Cape Breton Island. I ate a seafood dish and we all took a bite of each other's to share the experience. There I learnt that Govind was indeed gay. Jenny, "Shut it Govind, or I'll put a boot in your ass!" Me (jokingly), "He might enjoy that!" Govind, "I might just!"

Ten days after the Thanksgiving dinner (surprisingly we had a non-traditional non-turkey dinner), Jennifer organised a Halloween pumpkin party. In her apartment Hans, Yvonne, Christine, Kirsten, Govind, Hamoon, Jenny, Annie and myself carved pumpkins into assorted ghosts, ghouls and funnies before lighting them up with candles and leaving them on display overnight for all to be impressed. We ate pumpkin pie with cream and drank a homemade punch concocted by the American friends. An obscure green coloured goo was the result, but it had vodka in, so we all tried some out of politeness as much as to celebrate. Nobody died – hooray! Also in November I vaguely recollect a strippers' party that I was invited to and two young dancing girls came to perform for a whole room full of testosterone-filled males. Paul from Norway particularly enjoyed the ceremony, and Ulrich from Denmark. Hell, everyone enjoyed the ceremony; what a carry on that night! Later that night I met Katie from Canada, and it turned out that I had canoodled with the great-great-granddaughter of a Canadian Prime Minister, Mr Thompson, so there's something extraordinary!

Cora's breakfast bar always did great business with students, opening for breakfasts at 7am and going through for lunches until 3pm. You could equally buy a crepe with exotic fruit, fruit smoothies, or a full cooked breakfast; all brought to you in your very own booth with friends.....a perfect start to the day any day of the week, all at a reasonable rate. I went to Cora's three or four times that semester for a fabby brekky.

Two further trips occurred that semester. One to Cape Breton Island, October $8^{th} - 11^{th}$, and one to Prince Edward Island (PEI), Saturday 2nd / Sunday 3rd October, both in the North of Nova Scotia, a solid days driving to get there (3pm – 9pm). Both trips to me were a bit of a washout for one reason or another. For the trip to Cape Breton Island, there were three cars and we were supposed to communicate by cell (mobile) phone. But the reception was completely 'out', by the time the trip took place. I was driving with Nanneke, and the other two cars had already arranged their meeting place on the island. The arrangement was to keep in contact by phone, but as this couldn't happen, Nanneke and I made our very own travel itinerary around the island. We ended up walking and we even made it to a lovely beach as well. We saw some moose by the side of the road, so took some photographs. We drove to Baddeck, Sydney, Louisbourg and Cheticamp, staying in a motel, a seaside cabin, and a bed and breakfast in Sydney.

There I met another two travellers who were into making films, so we all went out for a Chinese roast duck meal, and then to the 'peanut bar' where the discarded peanut shells were thrown on the floor for the tender to clear at the end of the night. That evening a blues duo were jamming intensely in the bar, and we drank some beer before walking back to the B&B. The owner of the B&B was a burly ex-Royal Mounties officer, so everybody got up in time for a delicious breakfast the next morning! I managed to send some authentic Canadian maple syrup back home to mum for her birthday on 13th November from this trip, which was nice.

The second trip to PEI was with the Malaysian boys and American girls. We set off at 7am in order to catch the 10am ferry in the North. We made it and enjoyed an open topped ferry crossing on to PEI by lunchtime, for which we drove straight to Charlottetown and found a café to eat at. We booked tickets for the last night of the musical *Anne of Green Gables* (a Nova Scotian musical extremely popular with oriental girls as it represents the Canadian dream for a girl, or something along those lines). Annie is of Chinese descent.

After booking tickets we drove to a wonderfully quiet beach for a walk and played in the sand by a series of windmill-type structures, built for what purpose exactly I'm not so sure. Only today Jenny fell out with me…maybe my advances were unwelcome? So we walked with animosity between us. This rather altered the course of a happy day trip to an uncomfortable one. Must have been something I said, I'm sure!

The evening came and we returned to Charlottesville to eat pizza/falafel and watch the celebrated musical on the final night. Very diverting, I must admit. I enjoy live music and the dramatic storyline highlighted the excellent music too. So an opportune visit nonetheless. We drove back to Halifax, crossing the 'five mile bridge' (originally causing controversy with native islanders as the mainland was now attached to the island, so losing some of its authentic islandish state of being). We got home at around three o'clock in the morning, tired out, and we went straight to bed.

The high political event in that first semester was the visit of George W Bush (USA President) to Halifax to commend and extend his thanks to the people who had sheltered the diverted passengers from around the 9/11 disaster. Aeroplanes were diverted to Halifax from New York, and people needed a resting place for a while, so many Halifax residents offered a helping hand. The security forces even used Fenwick apartments as a look out tower, so men with rifles were scaling the building and looking out from the top floor.

The final international event that semester was to be a huge badminton tournament in the Sports centre. I would regularly swim there in the Olympic-sized pool, and play squash there with various partners. Also, Point Pleasant Park provided a popular spot to jog with colleagues. The shuttle bus would take ten minutes to drive onto campus, otherwise a twenty-minute walk would be necessary. I played doubles with a Chinese partner called Ron. We were beaten in the first round by two Norwegians. I enjoyed the game anyway, and stayed around to watch the whole tournament being played. Guess who won? Would you believe it, coming from the country of the highest living standards in the world, from Sweden....Peter and Sandra (a couple on and off the courts). They were on a one semester exchange and spent their Christmas holidays in Costa Rica. They had won five straight matches to win a cheque for CAD$100 and a reputation too. I loved Peter and Sandra very much and wish them all the very best for their futures and lives together (I hope).

December saw people busy with end-of-semester exams, Christmas arrangements, and a sad feeling that, for many, a one semester exchange was about to end. Annie had a friend visit all the way from Mexico and we walked together around the harbour and Halifax citadel where the old munitions and military relics remain visible, to this day. A changing of the guard occurs daily, as well, although I never witnessed the changing in Halifax (I later saw the changing of the guard in Quebec, but that's another story). My friend Chaz from Canada kept inviting me to play football with his friends, but I am no big fan of football. I remember inviting him to a Casino night with an international group...he is no big fan of Casinos, either. So we kept inviting each other and turning down each other. Anyhow, he was reading for an MBA and had been offered a professional internship in Europe the next year. I hope he was able to take that year. Jeff from Canada organized a December house party for all those still around. That was a mixed night where all sorts of emotion came to the fore amongst those present.

My written exams took place in the large sports hall, alongside hundreds of other students. I enjoyed writing as the questions from the Business in a Global Context paper allowed for creative extensions as well as hard facts. And I'm very good at creative extensions!

Whilst in Canada I opened up a Canadian Bank Account with the Bank of Montreal (BOM), although the other choices were equally valid, such as Scotia Bank or the Bank of Canada.

The most famous coffee shop outlet in Canada is without a doubt Tim Horton's. The equivalent of Starbucks in the UK, Tim Horton's was set up by an Ice-Hockey aficionado by the name of Tim Horton. He died, but to this day the whole charity side of the outlet is dedicated to teaching children how to play ice-hockey in Canada. We saw Canada beat the USA in the December world cup finals, 2004, so a big national celebration there! Our TV was no ordinary TV, as mentioned previously...more like a miniature home-cinema system. Thanks to Jesse and Dominic (the Fenwick mentors for International students) we all had full access to this system every day.

Major point of interest for December were the Christmas parades along Springbank Road. Carnival floats with dancers, singers, jugglers, harbour hoppers, Santa Claus, elves, reindeer, *the Grinch*, rescue choppers, police, Canadian Red Cross, ships and boats all passed by in the street. A sight to behold, even though the temperatures were down, and the queues for coffee exceptionally long (too long, in fact, to join). So we 'huddled' to keep warm. I wondered how the folk must have felt wearing their Scottish tartan kilts that night! One of my favourite nights out that semester was a by-product....we were supposed to go to 'The Palace', a nightclub, but I hated the whole atmosphere so left with two friends early. We went to a 24 hour Tim Horton's café and enjoyed mulled apple with a cinnamon bun and chatted amiably for a good 2 hours in that café. A great turning point to what was otherwise a dull night.

The final parties that semester were all out on the town. Spring Bank and Barrington Street provided the hub of activity for these. Pubs, bars and clubs such as Rogues' Roost (with Chris, Kate and Amanda), where a live band would often provide some cracking musical entertainment, Cheers bar (everybody), Pacifico or Rain nightclubs (I'm not a great fan of night clubs but occasionally I really enjoyed myself in a club), Dooly's American pool bar, My Father's Moustache, The Argyle, The Old Triangle (an Irish folksy bar where I ate lunch with Annie and her Mexican friend), or The Split Crow (a loud, youthful, rock-and-roll bar popular with service men/women as well as students) where a fight would often break out for no obvious reason. I spent my time there enjoying the music more than any other distraction. Richard the Swede got on well with me and told me of his dream to play football for a Swedish club one day. God speed your football feet, Richard - - - - - A cocktail bar provided pretty much the ultimate time together with these students before we moved on once again.

Christmas vacation – Atlantic International Christmas 2004

I had signed up with the University Christian Fellowship to the 'Atlantic International Christmas 2004'. After the other students had left I walked to the Student Union where the transport bus awaited us, 12pm Wednesday, 22nd December. There I chatted with Desmond from Ethiopia and Kayhan from Iran. My bus journey was relatively quiet as we drove to Sackville, New Brunswick. We were registered to stay in Mount St Alison University lodgings. As it happens, this Christmas holiday away from home changed my life in three massive ways. 1) I learnt that it *was* possible to spend an entire Christmas away from home and survive the experience, 2) I met my then girlfriend (Taisya) whom I dated for 10 months afterwards, and 3) I felt closer to God than ever before. Being a Christian holiday, we had a lot of social and communal activities, church on Christmas Day, and an entirely integral ethic going on the whole time as well.

There were more people there than I can remember now, but I will try, anyhow. So again, a wholesome multicultural social experience, I met Abebaw and Desmond from Ethiopia, Victor, Djerri, Steve, Andu and Uzo from Nigeria, Jim, Josh (a loud and rude boy), Luke, Tim, Dave "don't take wooden nickels", Adam (and his Dad) from Canada, Val from Malaysia, Mike and his girlfriend from China, Stephanie and Katriona from Germany (the latter of whom had an affair with Andu), Gordon Flowerdew – musical father of Collum, Mark, Adele, and Saatchi (looked after by a Canadian girl Heather)-, Tanya from Mexico, Anmol from India, Kayhan from Iran, Taya from Russia, and Sarah, one of the Canadian organisers of the holiday.

Every day we would dine communally with breakfast at 8am in a central canteen area, lunch at 1pm, and dinner at 7pm. The food was served by catering assistants and we would take our own trays to the respective seating area.

Our first activity was ten-pin bowling and ice-skating…not at the same time, you understand, but on the same day, anyhow. I went purposefully anti-clockwise round the skating rink whilst everyone else went clockwise. Method in my madness? To take lots of pictures of people skating forwards, rather than of their behinds.

We had plenty of snow all the time there; fun for building snowballs, snowmen (or snow-people to be politically correct) and general winter atmosphere. Even to walk between buildings proved a real challenge and shock to the system some days. It was really that cold. Brrrrrrrrr!!!!!

Many buildings there were sporting Canadian flags atop them which blew patriotically in the wind. A splendid sight to behold, I found. One afternoon I found myself participating in some weird circular dancing method, clapping my hands two-a-plenty. We all walked round and round to the rhythm of the music and kept in time, and kept our places. Fun nonetheless. The Christmas Choir would rehearse every morning, of which I took part as a bass/baritone voice. I enjoyed this singing component, must admit.

One night we had an International Banquet and an International Fashion Show. For the banquet I cooked 'British bangers 'n' mash' and for the fashion show I sat watching as the splendid African and Asian costumes took *way* precedence in the proceedings. Other dishes included Ethiopian Goat Curry, Indian Samosas, Chinese Chow Mein, and Canadian meat.

I shared a room with Kayhan, until he became poorly and broke into a fever, so I changed rooms at this point and went downstairs to a single room. Poor fellow, nice guy, and fortunately he recovered well enough within two days to continue with the vacation. Whilst listening to my portable radio one night in this room I learned about the tragic Malaysian Tsunami which killed so many people.

This leads me to the Talent night itself. Here people gave of themselves readily. On the talent night, Kayhan taught everybody the Farsi alphabet. A table tennis tournament had been going on throughout the duration of the holiday. On talent night I faced Abebaw in the grand final. It turns out that Ethiopia beat the UK at table tennis, so Abebaw won the t-shirt – just! Also on talent night there was music, comedy, drama, and a guy called Steve (Canadian) doing very funny impersonations. I sang Elton John's *'Your Song'* on Organ, with guitar and tabla drummer accompanying. People seemed to appreciate this, so I even got an applause, even though the top note was missing from the keyboard.

The village pond was frozen solid, so we made good use of this to skate on and play 'ice football' for a while. I was somewhat nervous about going on the ice as I had seen movies where kids fall right into the icy cold water through the ice. Nobody fell through here, though. Luckily for all, the pond was solid through and through.

Christmas Day was really nice, for want of a better word. We woke up in the morning to receive especially selected Christmas stockings, jam-packed full of goodies and surprises. I had slept in by mistake this morning so was the last person to receive a stocking. No worries. There was a wonderful carol service in Sackville church and we were all invited to walk to a local family's house and share some Christmas banter with the family. A really wonderful way to spend the day itself. Christmas dinner was back in the communal hall, where a special turkey feast had been prepared for us all to enjoy. And enjoy it I did. Following the meal, Anmol dressed as Santa and distributed one main present to each person there. I received a portable radio system which I listened to often until the wiring went faulty on it after a year or so. A great gift for my travels. Outstanding stuff, AIC2004!

My final memory of this holiday was Taya's birthday on 26th December; we all were invited to go square-dancing with professionals leading the proceedings. Everybody partnered up (I with Taisya) and arranged themselves into small groups, whilst the MC maintained our sense of direction, giving clear instructions what foot to place where, when to do so, and how to keep up with the rhythm. The professionals even gave us all a very explicit demonstration themselves, then cleared the floor for all us rabble to have a dance.

So, fun and games all around, and then time to pack our bags and return to Halifax. The bus was bombarded with an assault of snowballs as we drove away again at 10:30am Tuesday, 28th December. Those naughty Canadian boys sure knew how to see off honoured guests. We returned to Halifax, and I agreed to meet up with Taya sometime soon before she was given a lift home to Acadia University, Wolfville. Sure enough we continued to meet throughout the second semester and our relationship continued on into the Summer holidays 2005 where she visited me in England before flying to Calgary University to read for a Computer Science Master's degree. Our relationship ended soon after this, but I truly treasure the time we spent together, and the memories are happy and will be with me forever.

*On into New Year 2004/05…..*Taisya visited me in Halifax to spend New Year here. Other students from AIC2004 also came out to the radio festival in Town Hall Square that cold (but not freezing) night. We 'saw in' the New Year by drinking in an English bar called Maxwell's Plum; Rickard's Honey Brown Ale (Taya's first taste of the stuff), eating peanuts and cracking a good yarn. By midnight we were all out in the festival arena for the fireworks ceremony. That was by far the most exciting Christmas/New Year experience in my adult life, until 2008 when I remet Christina back home in Scarborough, U.K. That year was truly different for me.

Semester Two: January 2005 – April 2005

That year the new recruits all came in. We had Rick, Myrte, Rosie, Anne, and Mariella from the Netherlands, Anne and Hannah from Germany, Axel, Anna, and Sarah from Sweden, Mario from Mexico, Andreas from Denmark, Fiona and Jolene from Australia, Gabriel and Alex from Mexico, and I made friends with Chaz from Canada on another floor. He kept inviting me to play football – one of my least favourite pastimes. Also I made a Canadian friend whom I had met hitchhiking around Cape Breton Island in October – John Gaudi – who was beginning an internship with a Canadian television corporation in Halifax. Swedish Richard and Danish Lotte both commissioned me to hug Amy for them this New Year!

In January my modules also changed. Now I was reading Logistics Management (Pat Bohan simultaneously teaching, reading for a Master's degree, working in Halifax Docks, and rearing children of his own who, on occasion, came into the lecture theatre to see their daddy), Production/Operations Management (Hugh Gassmann – didn't like the module or the professor…too mathematical for me), New Venture Creation (Ed Leech – we were given free will to choose our own projects, so I made a series of surveys to dispense around local coffee shops in Halifax, and studied/analysed the results), and International Business (my absolutely preferred module by choice, with Don Patton, ex-Canadian ambassador to Indonesia). Two notable events were a Logistics field trip to the docks for an education, and a discussion on a book by Robert Rubin, with Don Patton. I enjoyed these two experiences.

On the whole I was happy with my workload, as well. Anyhow, the snow was high by the end of the month so we decided to take advantage of this fact and go skiing, especially because school had been *snowed off* for 10 days! Ski Wentworth is a 'local' Nova Scotian mountain range and Charles, Matt, Amy, Anna, Myrte, Andreas, Sarah, Anne 1 and Anne 2, Mario, myself, Liz, Jolene and Gabriel all took off on skis, Friday, 4th February. Funnily some of the routes had extraordinary names to them such as: "Pugwash", "Gooey", "Feffie Weffie", "Robins", "Giggletree", "Gambol", "Garden Path", or "Embree", but the names did not detract from the pleasure of skiing. I began on the nursery slopes after many years non-practice, but soon gravitated to the proper slopes up the ski lifts with the others. Terrific, great fun, I was really glad to be there!

The very first evening that we were all together that semester we had a communal meal in the dining area. I remember particularly Jolene, Myrte, Anna, Sarah, Amy, Anne, Mario, Hannah, Andreas, Rick, Matt, Alex and Gabriel. We all sat around acclimatising and getting to know one another from scratch. No mean feat by anyone's standards. Another noteworthy event in January has to be the *Frat party* in a Canadian home. They had their own basement bar downstairs and played loud music. For entertainment there was table tennis and darts. I enjoyed myself that night, as did most others. The photographs demonstrate our happiness.

The Green Dragon

Most weekends I would see Taisya, either I would visit by bus to Wolfville, or she would visit by bus to Halifax. We would often spend our time walking together in the parks, in the snow, or sipping fresh coffee in the local coffee shops. This was a very welcome activity in the freezing cold winter days. Our favourite café in Halifax was called 'Uncommon Grounds', of which there were three. Also, my survey spree enabled me to discover many more coffee shops than by purely passive consumerism. I loved going to the cafés, and to me, that remains a 'best bit' – so much so that I coined a notion that one day I would run my own coffee shop/café back in the UK. I especially appreciated the fair-trade coffee, and any in-house bakeries where fresh breads and pastries would be baked on a daily basis early in the morning, then put out for sale. That combined smell of fresh roast coffee and baking is just wonderful to smell when you're hungry and cold, stepping in from the street into the coffee house.

February saw numerous other festivals, parties and celebrations. We had Anne's birthday, an International concert, a Keg party, a pyjama party, an evening watching the NFL Superbowl on the cinematic TV, and the month's highlight – a trip to Montreal and Toronto for five days. First, Anne's 21st birthday was to be formidable. We set up a barbecue on the patio outdoors (sheltered from any winds) and wore silly hats. Also, Charles had obtained a pair of walkie-talkies. As he was speaking, an unexpected frequency was picked up, and a complete stranger began to sing to us all. We took it in turns to sing back which was hilarious. We ate Dutch and German food that evening as well as standard barbecued sausage…Deeelicious.

Second, the International Concert; for this I had been secretly rehearsing with Mario. I played piano/lead vocals and Mario guitar/backing vocals. We learnt the songs *"He ain't heavy, he's my brother"*, by the Hollies, and *"Imagine"* by John Lennon. In front of approximately 400 people we performed these numbers. It went well. Our secret practice had paid off. Also that evening we saw some Brazilian Capuera dancers – a form of non-contact martial art where the participants make all the manoeuvres at a steadily increasing pace to the rhythm of drums. It got really fast but everyone seemed in full control of themselves...phew! Also, some Afro-American hip-hop dancers performed a raunchy number. The Mexicans serenaded the audience on guitars (including Gabriel and Alex), and a lone Chinese ballerina performed a whole dance routine, stunningly so.

That semester I was keeping in touch with Ruth and Paul, sometimes catching the ferry across to Dartmouth to help them build a fence or the barn or sometimes to go and chat with Taya. In the first semester around October time I had taken my Malaysian friends there as well to visit. Paul showed us his rifles, and Ellie had grown so much from being a tiny little puppy dog into a full grown bitch. She even peed on the Fenwick carpets at an October party, for which she was pardoned unconditionally. She was only an irresponsible pup at the time.

The Keg party coincided with an American Football match on television...an NFL Superbowl contest. And the *pyjama party* was Hannah's big idea. Contrary to my usual practice of sleeping nude I wore t-shirt and boxer shorts. My honest revelation made everyone laugh out loud when I told them.

The month's big event...1pm Friday, 18th February, we caught the train and rode for 16 hours to Montreal, passing some very Franglais sounding towns eg 'Bienvenue à Truro'. On the journey we all crammed into one carriage. That is: Axel, Anna, Myrte, Mariella, Sarah, Matt, Anne, Fiona, Andreas, Naomi, Mario, Anne, Hannah, me, Jolene, and others too. In Montreal we arrived in time for breakfast so having dropped off our luggage at the Youth Hostel, we visited a local bagel bar 'St Viateur'. Couldn't help but notice that the menus were equally in French and English. So my bagel with cream cheese and sliced tomato was doubly interesting. After breakfast we went walk-about and headed up Mount Royale (the origin of the name 'Montreal') where from the top the cityscape vista is just remarkable, looking out over the corporate Banks of Montreal, skyscrapers, city architecture old and new, and the watery bay area.

The Green Dragon

During our visit to Montreal we called in the indoor shopping mall where ice skaters skated on the arena, and we called in the Notre Dame Cathedral, which is very French and Catholic in aura. Outside of this were queuing horses and wagons to escort tourists around the city. All over the city we could see adverts of <u>Art Vista</u> advertising Montreal Jazz, as the huge festival takes place in July, famous all over the world. Schwartz's famous smoked meat café did not go unnoticed. I queued there for half an hour to get my taste of this celebrated gammon accompanied by pickled gherkin and washed down with Dr Pepper soft drink. The Swedish couple with whom I shared the moment were to split up within two months. One morning we visited the modern art gallery, where John acted as our Canadian host. Later that evening we collaborated in determining a social gathering and the agreement was 'Upstairs' jazz bar (ironically this is a basement bar), but the venue was sold out so we went to an English style pub called the 'Cock and Bull'. There a superb guitar player was jamming on folksy-blues riffs. I did not know the hooks he used, but the melody lines really cut through making the evening a splendid occasion. China town in Montreal also received a visit and we dined one evening in a Chinese restaurant.

The final visit in Montreal was to the Olympic Stadium built for the 1976 Summer Games. We climbed on board the sky train and ascended the Olympic tower. The day was extremely snowy so the proper Olympic village view was somewhat hazy. The records provided interesting reading in the reception museum, and the swimming pool was still open for public usage. I felt inclined to go for a dip but had not brought my trunks with me.

On Monday, 21st February we caught the train to Toronto, which unlike Montreal, seemed purely corporate; lots of big commercial conglomerates, banks, companies, big businesses etc. We lodged in the Global Village for Backpackers youth hostel. Very modern, with their own bar, internet access, clean bed linen, washrooms, pool table and open mic night where performers could get up and sing if they wished to do so. No complaints about the hostel apart from breakfast being a bit sparse - one bagel with coffee and jam. No other options were available.

We visited Planet Hollywood where I placed my hand in the hand-print of Steven Segal. We visited the Toronto Stock Exchange, but exchanged no shares; I knew that Glenn Gould recorded in Toronto during his lifetime, playing Bach on piano; the judge's court house received a visit from us, although not in the capacity of cops and criminals---mere tourists! We climbed the CN tower by lift and enjoyed the view of Lake Ontario on one side, and Toronto City on the other. I bought a photograph of our group standing on the glass-bottomed height of Toronto CN Tower with a drop to the ground of hundreds of feet. Also we visited the Toronto NASDAQ stock exchange HQ. Although we were only able to set foot in the visitors 'lounge' the atmosphere was very upbeat through and through.

The main highlight of the Toronto visit was the trip to Niagara Falls via the Ice-wine vineyards. *Inniskillin* produce annual harvests of Ice wine and sell it by the narrow bottle full. They call it ice wine because the grapes are harvested when still frozen in the winter time. This produces a concentrated, sweet flavour. The cold wind comes off Lake Ontario and blows across the vineyards, as they are on flat terrain. The Falls were icy cold and even the tunnels beneath were iced through so one could not see through all the windows. Some students went out in a helicopter to get a better view. I stayed on the ground but got extremely cold and wet from the severe wind and icy spray.

And this was pretty much the trip to Montreal and Toronto. We caught the train to both places from Halifax and then came back by aeroplane from Toronto to Halifax International airport, returning home by taxicab, Saturday, 26th February. Also this day we celebrated Matt's 21st birthday.

That brings me to March and April 2005. That semester there were several notable couples who partnered up. First and foremost: Axel and Anna (long-term partners who had been together since the age of 16), also Andreas and Hannah (who I believe are still together five years later), Mario and German Anne, Charles and Sarah, Matt and Beverley, and myself and Taisya. The whole semester seemed together like that in a closely-knit community. Saturday, 19th March, saw Amy's 21st masked birthday party.

Some Sundays a small group would while away the time in Point Pleasant Park. One weekend I was there sunbathing with Rick, Matt, Sarah, Axel and Andreas whilst others were walking their dogs, jogging, playing Frisbee and so on. I enjoyed the weekend farmer's market with Taisya. On a Saturday morning the local farmers would set up their stalls on the ground floor of the Keith's Nova Scotian Brewery. The full range of organic produce was terrific, all the vegetables, meats, dairy products, fruits, vegan foods amassed to quite an impressive display.

German Anne organised a cocktail party at which Carlos got friendly with Hannah, Mario enjoyed Moosehead beer from a can, and I revelled in the music choice being played.

April's highlight has to be the second journey to Cape Breton Island in a double convoy of two cars from Wednesday 20th – Saturday 23rd. A Buddhist monastery called Gampo Abbey complete with a shrine of wisdom can be found in a remote spot. Incidentally, even to get there is a lovely three mile drive, off any main route. We stayed at the Cabot Trail Hostel and learnt of local walking routes such as the Skyline Trail, which we walked seeing moose and eagles along the way. We walked extra carefully so as not to scare the moose into charging us as they reputedly are known to do at times. Much of the Skyline Trail is lined with a boardwalk to make walking easier and drier underfoot. I wondered whoever had the time of day to go ahead and build such a lengthy, and yet entirely remote, boardwalk. It was a privilege to be able to use the walk, nonetheless.

The car ride was full of gaffs *en voyage* as we travelled. An iPod and walkie-talkie connected the two vehicles, with Charles and Matt in charge of the speaking. We shared the driving; in our car I shared with Sarah. In a coastal and remote spot I noticed a sign for a "Whale Interpretive Centre" so this left me wondering how any human being could be employed to speak, or even interpret, whale-speak. It was closed when we arrived so I never got to find out. Also, the seagulls flew proud and reminded me of Richard Bach's famous book *'Jonathan Livingstone Seagull'*. In the hostel we shared some food, ale, jokes, and enlightening conversation. A café near Baddeck fed us on our travels and I am almost certain that a descendant of Alexander Graham Bell was having his lunch *en famille*. His beard resembled him, and his portly belly too.

As we discovered numerous remote and tranquil locations we ended up paddling barefoot, clambering on rocks, walking on beaches, throwing rocks/stones hard onto the ice to try and smash it open (the ice floe came in direct from the North Atlantic and many seabirds would perch themselves on the ice as it floated on the ocean surface). A quad bike bezzed about on one beach as we watched for a moment.

This trip was breath-taking and <u>changed my life completely for the better</u>. In complete contrast to October's trip in semester one, everybody bonded and there was no falling out during the space of our five day sojourn. I was sad to leave Cape Breton Island this time, and feel that I left a part of myself on the remote island in some quiet spot.

By the time May came round and final exams were over, people were beginning to feel a bit low, realising that the whole exchange phenomenon was soon to draw to a close. At the final party Joseph drank too much whisky, so I gave him a glass of salt water to drink. He threw up and then drank LOTS of fresh water to compensate for the nasty taste. Magnus from Norway got talking to me about impulsive behaviour. I really enjoyed this conversation as it gave me a chance to explore some psychological phenomena such as nature/nurture and logic/stability vs impulse/excitement. I do believe that life is full of paradigms so the paradigm of impulse was good to talk about.

One by one people left for the airport, and I saw them off with Taisya. Fortunately I was staying on to go travelling independently in June so loads of useful items were left behind for me to use while I remained in Fenwick, and food too. Taya had graduated from Acadia University by now and came to live with me for two weeks before flying home to Russia to spend the summer with her family. We visited the Kejimkujik National Park on a day excursion, and in between completing my final exams (I really struggled with Production/Operations management) and travelling independently I continued training for the Halifax 10km race on Sunday, 22nd May 8:45am. The actual event was a full marathon, but the weather was appalling with strong winds and torrential rain. This did not prevent everybody from turning out to run the race anyway. I saw the start whilst listening to Eye of the Tiger on the overhead sound system. This fired me up and filled me with inspiration, 'I should run a full marathon myself!', before I ran the 10km in one hour straight. During this period I still lived in Fenwick apartments and kept in contact with the Iranian brothers Kayhan and Ali Mahdavi. One day they invited me to the Students Union with their friends to watch the European Cup final football match. Liverpool won the title having come back and turned round a 3-0 deficit at half time.

On the evenings before Taya flew home we often went out into town. One evening we visited Stainer's Jazz bar, as the live Atlantic Jazz festival was going on there. We heard a quartet playing: alto saxophone, drums/percussion, double bass, and electric keyboard/vocals. I thought they were phenomenal. By this point the prospect of making it to the Montreal Jazz Festival in July really appealed to me. Also, we dined out at Chives one night, a posh restaurant in town on Barrington Street. We literally whiled away the entire evening together wining, dining and then sitting on the comfy sofa, just chatting away about whatever - my favourite occupation at the time! The last night together we cracked open a bottle of Organic red Zinfandel wine and got merry and silly together. We realised it may be the last time we were to meet, were it not for our cunning plan to travel around the U.K. in August. Taya caught the plane home the very next morning and returned "to Russia with love". I drove to Springfield where I visited the Anne Murray Centre and bought some goodies for my friend and now running partner David Goodwin back home in the U.K.

Independent travel June/July 2005

With tickets booked to fly from Halifax to Vancouver on June 4th, then to travel gradually East on the Greyhound coach via Edmonton, Calgary, the Rockies, Thunder Bay; to fly from Thunder Bay to Ottawa; train to Montreal for Independence Day and the Jazz Festival, then train home to Halifax where Ruth and Paul would meet me for a night and take me to the airport-home; this takes us into my personal adventure across Canada. NB a strong theme across Canada at this time of year is Jazz! The main festival is in Montreal but artists literally fly to play in each venue, one after the other. More on this as we go along.

Fortunately for me Taisya had made friends with a Russian taxi driver before she went home, and as it transpires he decided to be my friend as well. At 5am on my departure morning he arrived at Fenwick to collect me and drive me to the airport. Only, because he was our friend he refused payment, so an otherwise $30 taxi ride was free of charge for me - *"Bolshoi Spasiba, Miguel!"*

Flying via Toronto, where I had to change planes with a 2 hour wait, I arrived in Vancouver that same day. The in-flight movie this time was called 'St Ralph' about a 14-year-old-boy at a Catholic school who ran the Senior Boston marathon and came -----2nd (just!!) I think it was fiction, as no one younger than 18 years can officially run a senior marathon anyway, but I thoroughly enjoyed watching the film; actually it inspired me to run one myself later (Paris, April 2006). But that is another story for another page some other time.

Once in the city of Vancouver I made my way to the Main Street CN hostel where I had booked in previously online. They have a public transport system of *sky-cars* in Vancouver. That is,

The Green Dragon

cabins on rails like the London Underground, only going above the city surface in the air - pleasant to view the city from as you travel. I walked and booked in to the hostel by tea time. First things first – have a shower and purchase some food and drink to relax with after a long flight. In my case I found a local sushi bar (there are many in Vancouver) and drank Saki to wash it down. I was very intrigued by the way that the trays of raw fish go round in little boats on the conveyor belt. Diners simply pick and choose as the 'boats' go past. Being in Vancouver for five days, I had plenty of time to travel over the next few days. On day one I joined a tour bus with a guide on board pointing out all the sights of the city. We went round China town (lots of current day problems with junkies, heroin users, and drug pushers here), the marina with yachts a plenty, Granville market also by the water's edge, full of interesting shops to buy luscious goods in. Fresh produce was imported daily in the huge and diverse fruit, vegetable, fish, and other food stores. In addition to this the music was live by the water's edge, so as I sat munching my lunch, Leonard Cohen's 'Hallelujah' accompanied the moment. Indeed this was a hallelujah moment; I could not find a better word for it on reflection.

We drove into and around Stanley Park where I saw native Indian culture totem poles. The top bird with 'wings outstretched' indicates a peaceful village where visitors are welcome. A top bird with 'wings by the side' indicates a village at unrest so visitors are to be warded off. Also in Stanley Park we stopped at the 'Wishing Tree', a giant redwood with a huge hollow carved out of it. The legend is that if you stand there with closed eyes you get to make a wish. I did so gladly! A mermaid out in the water is used as an indicator of high tide, ie when the water is up to her foot then you will know. She is a statue by day and by night you would just have to see for yourself. As I walked back later that day I felt inspired to stop off at a karaoke bar, so I gave a rendition of two numbers "Alive and kicking" by Simple Minds, and "It's not unusual" by Tom Jones. God only knows why I chose these two, but there you are.

Walking round town later, I discovered the Art Gallery where Rodin was being exhibited. So being a curious art appreciator I payed a visit here. A highlight for me in Vancouver was to go to the Sport Memorabilia museum where all Canada's Sporting and Olympic heroes are commemorated. One guy in particular was "Terry Fox", who contracted cancer of the leg and had it amputated. He then proceeded to run across Canada with a prosthetic leg, in the form of daily marathons for weeks and months on end. He got as far as Thunder Bay where he collapsed. The support crew drove him to hospital where it was discovered his cancer had spread into the rest of his body. Soon after, he died and was nominated a national hero for his courage to carry on. They played St Elmo's fire, which was Terry's most motivating tune, in the museum.

On talking with a room-mate at the youth hostel, we agreed that the Montmartre café just 5km up the road was well worth spending time at, a bohemian French style café with live poetry and music to sample whilst enjoying some refreshment. I arrived, and a lovely waitress named Courtney looked after me that evening, even drawing directions to all my request stops in Vancouver. That evening a French piano-playing songwriter named Samuel played his own material and I enjoyed drinking G&T whilst flirting with Courtney. I even went back one more time before I left Vancouver to say goodbye. Who knows, maybe we will meet again one day?

On day three I hired out a bicycle from the hostel and made my own tour of the city. Very beautiful with the Rocky mountains on one side and the Pacific Ocean on the other, with modern Vancouver's skyscrapers interspersed in between. An extremely clean and lucrative city all in all. I would love to go back there one day and be there all over again. I returned to Stanley Park and enjoyed the cooling rafters of a café there. But a lifeguard told me off en route for cycling in front of his cabin rather than behind it. In fact, to make his point, he chased after me and insisted that I get off and push my bike past. Comical? Annoying? Both maybe. I returned to my totem poles and to the famous wishing tree to make one more wish there. My guess is that it worked, but that would be telling! The wish, that is.

Grouse Mountain, the local Vancouver mountain looming over the entire city was next on my list. So off I travelled by ferry boat, bus and cable car to get there. I paid my fare for a day pass and to my delight found myself face to face with wolves and grizzly bears (enclosed by an electric fence), and watched a live falconry display, too. There were giant redwood trees with artistic carvings in them, the city scape below and a world famous lumberjack show to enjoy as two men battled it out sawing, climbing, axe-throwing and log rolling. One slipped and hurt his groin, but he will live anyhow for another day to continue his show. I got lost at one point as I walked off the beaten track and nearly fell down a cliff side. Fortunately I kept my balance and made it back to the pathway once again.

When in Vancouver, there is one activity that all tourists feel compelled to do – Whale Watching. I went out in a boat one morning with a group of ten others (not including the pilot and tour guide) and saw several pods of Killer Whales. I don't recall the temperature, but it was June so summer heat was present, although there was an ocean wind to contend with, and my hat remained firmly strapped on by my chin before we set out. Also this day I saw some eagles fishing by the water's edge. I really had a sense of profound, peaceful privilege being here at this point in my life. A very beautiful place in the world, indeed.

My last night in Vancouver, I went and sat in a Portuguese restaurant and enjoyed a plateful of liver and mashed potatoes with onion. I drank a local brew to wash this down. Plus a Seattle coffee shop the next morning before catching the bus. Not actually in the USA, mind, but they like their neighbouring city so much that a whole coffee shop is named after it. This was my Vancouver time over now, and so I caught the Greyhound bus east to Calgary, next. We stopped at Edmonton on the way, as well as numerous other spots. On the bus I chatted with a few people about their own travel experiences in Canada and elsewhere in the world.

Over 30 hours on the same bus is not anybody's idea of fun, even though driving through the Rockies could be very beautiful at times. Calgary was to be my next choice stop with a three-day adventure lined up in the Rocky mountains - horse-back riding, hiking, and white-water rafting. Before this, though, a day exploring Calgary on foot. I got off the Greyhound bus at the station and put my rucksack into a locker there. Then as I was wondering which way best to go into town from the taxi rank, a nearby woman was also wondering the same thing. We got talking whether to share a taxi, but she then said that she knew Calgary well so we should walk together and she would show me some of the sights there. So we took the half hour walk into town from the bus station and she began to tell me her life story, how her boyfriend back in her home city had beaten her and emptied the joint bank account of all funds. Ah!? Then she proceeded to tell me of her sister whom she had come to visit in Calgary, as she lived here and would offer her work for the time being…..cash in hand. We kept walking and began looking for the 'Cecil Hotel' where she worked. When finally we arrived there we sat and had a beer together, and I began to look around with eyes wide open and what did I see? Never before had I set foot in such a seedy dive for a place with the most slutty wenches in the world. I'm convinced to this day that the hotel was some sort of brothel for working women in Calgary, so I made my excuses and went off looking for a pair of hiking boots for the Rockies expedition ahead.

'Randy' met me in a 4x4 truck at the bus station and drove me for three hours to base camp in the mountains. Day one was to be horseback riding, day two hiking, and day three white water rafting. My horse was called 'Buzz' and was getting on slightly in years by now. Our group of four was led by an authentic cowboy from the ranch. We stopped for lunch, cooking hotdogs on sharp sticks, over an open fire in the woods. The scenery was just amazing…vast forests and mountains in all directions. Lakes, waterways, glacial rivers with crystal-clear waters in all the valleys. A freshening sense of spiritual karma struck me whilst there. A sense that everything was going to be OK, no matter what.

The Green Dragon

We rode all day, then came back to the ranch before nightfall where I showered in an obscure but warm shower device. You would have to see the photograph to believe it. A black cat had recently given birth to a litter of kittens in the ranch barn as well, so we got to witness these. I was living in a log cabin in the Rocky Mountains for 3 nights. My dream had come true! During the day's hiking, Randy, my tour guide, had come prepared for bears. We went into Calgary on my arrival and visited the outdoor shop and then bought pizza in a bar, with a beer to drink. Very communal, I'll say. During the trek we had to cross an ice-cold stream at the top of a huge waterfall. To keep our boots dry we took them off and crossed bare foot. My blisters got a real surprise. We found a cute little alcove near another waterfall for lunch. Also, during the day's trek we saw beavers and ducks swimming in a beautiful lake. Finally, here was the white-water rafting. A Canadian company called *"Creative Concepts"* had decided to undertake a team-building exercise together. As it happens, this was the same day's rafting as mine. Great stuff in actual fact – I got to raft with a proper team of people in two big boats. We took a paddle each and steered our way down stream through some really turbulent waters. At one point we rafted up to land and jumped into this freezing water off the rocks. Personally, I loved this swimming about bit! The CEO of the company was very young; only early 30s I recall.

After this jaunt in the mountains, Randy dropped me off back in Calgary where I stayed for one week in L'Auberge Chez Nous 149 5th Avenue S E, and had two main projects to visit…a) the Olympic Stadium, and b) Calgary Zoo. The River Bow was in flood at that time, so many tow-paths were fenced off officially. As I had borrowed my walking boots from the University Outdoor Pursuits Centre, I returned them and told them about my blisters. They apologised. How very British, I thought! By the local river-banks I saw snakes, beavers and loads of gophers. They were swarming everywhere. At the Olympic Stadium, from the 1980s Winter Olympics, I saw the ski jump, luge, bobsleigh, and skeleton run. Also, some great artwork presented a very international theme to the place.

At Calgary Zoo I had the privilege of seeing the following animals: tigers, warthogs, ponies, black bears, assorted monkeys, Indian elephants, antelopes, owls, gorillas, pink flamingos, llamas, crocodile/alligators, cookaburra birds, other exotic birds, kangaroos with joeys, emus, zebras, giraffes, lions, porcupines, boa constrictors, hippopotami, reindeer, eagles, mountain goats, geese, bison, dinosaur sculptures, red pandas, and squirrels.

These two attractions are all I can remember of Calgary, other than visiting various eateries, and musical events, eg the jazz festival, where I saw several artists perform here, too. The world famous Calgary Stampede is in July so I was not able to see this event as I was due to travel on by that time. So, next stop Thunder Bay (by Greyhound once again). This journey took a real long time. All I remember is that I was sitting next to an Indian girl called Sarah talking in French. She was on the way to Montreal, myself to Thunder Bay.

When we eventually arrived in Thunder Bay the question arose – how to get to the hostel from the bus station? As it was an extra 15km away or so I was not too certain how best to do this. Fortunately for me, there was a change of bus drivers and the first driver offered me a lift in his car all the way to the hostel. We discussed some of the Greyhound bus service driving stratagems, such as stopping at every level crossing, and how often rest-breaks are deemed necessary. Anyhow, we got there, and so I made it to the International Youth Hostel at Thunder Bay.

Here, Lloyd and his wife managed the hostel. I met a Japanese girl called Wakako, two French travellers called Robert and Danielle, a Thunder Bay native called Bronson who had colonic cancer – heavily into writing literature, a Burmese refugee working at the hostel for Lloyd, and a Canadian cyclist who beat me at chess – shucks! Lloyd's daughter Gail managed another youth hostel elsewhere in town so we kept bumping into each other throughout my stay. We were shown the local river, which proved perfect for bathing in, jumping into from rocks, and generally taking a dip. Also, a waterfall caused consternation whether to jump into it or not. I chose not to, as the water was running pretty hard, it seemed to me.

Lloyd had all his visitors make a sign for their native city, so I made one for York (Eboracum), 7767km east from here. Surprisingly a few other Yorkshire signs existed such as Hunton (Yorkshire Dales), Leeds (West Yorkshire), and other UK places such as Newcastle, Durham, Devon and Cornwall. Being a Christian man Lloyd took us all to his local church one Sunday where the Minister made a special announcement for the English traveller! I told him the bus ride was a long one.

On a general drive about town we saw the Marina on Lake Superior with all the boats, the Thunder Bay indoor golf driving range, wild grizzly bears on a dumping ground (I cautiously took some photos without getting too close), Terry Fox's memorial at the point where he collapsed on his marathon trans-Canadian run, and last but not least, a piece of municipal land owned by Lloyd in the shore front gardens, where he planted a commemorative tree for me before I left and called the conifer the "Jamie tree", telling me to check it next time I pass by Thunder Bay! I certainly intend to do so. Next morning Lloyd drove me to the airport where I said goodbye to Wakako, and continued on to Ottawa.

I got a bus into town and then walked to my hostel, the 'Backpackers Inn', 203 York Street, in the capital city. I found Ottawa to be extremely political in nature, the seat of government, Houses of Parliament, Prime Minister's home (then Paul Martin), and plenty of war memorials dedicated to the heroes who fought in Europe earlier in the 20th Century.

On my first night I met an American Jamie and a Brazilian Daniella. All three of us went out to a restaurant for dinner before roaming around a very hot, humid Ottawa, sight-seeing. Guess what?? The Jazz Festival had also made it to Ottawa…I just had to buy a ticket to a gig. I saw Diana Krall (Elvis Costello's wife), singing her own jazzy song-material, and two folksy musicians Bella Fleck (Banjo) and John Ponty (Violin). Their atmosphere was just phenomenal, I could have swum in it. Instead I sat in the park eating a crepe and chatting with a strange woman.

Canadian Independence day was soon coming, so a fellow group of young travellers also at the hostel tried to persuade me to stay with them in Ottawa for the festival ceremonies, but alas my ticket to Montreal was booked already. Incidentally, Wakako had made it to Ottawa too. She stayed in Ottawa for a further two years teaching in a school and studying as a student simultaneously. The connection from Lloyd in Thunder Bay was a good one and I will always remember this throughout my life. So, the train to Montreal…

…L'Auberge de Jeunesse, my French hostel in Central Montreal, 103 Mackay Street, was perhaps the best quality hostel that I stayed in throughout my stay; I'm glad that I had pre-booked, as the hostel was teeming when I arrived. Fortunately for me I had my own place to stay and the hostel management put on a guided tour of Montreal especially with a view to showing visitors Old Town for Independence Day. I recall meeting lots of Chinese travellers that night, Tim from Australia, Wolfgang from Germany, Janine and Peter from Switzerland, a lady from New York City, and the Canadian hosts who exhibited a whole-lot-of-fun character. The fireworks were fantastic that night, and we enjoyed a beverage whilst listening to live bands playing.

I took myself off on a personal walkabout of Montreal and revisited Mont Royale, un très beau panorama. Also, a French bookstore provoked a significant cultural interest for me, although I opted not to purchase any books. Maybe next time I pass by a French book store I may buy some French literature. Actually, that's a promise! I returned to the Montreal Olympic Stadium where the weather was no longer snowy, so I got a proper look round this time (compared with February). I visited an animal sanctuary too, where I saw turkeys, sting rays, tuna fish, sea vegetables, pelicans and penguins. The penguins made me think of the feature film Happy Feet (or vice versa for those

The Green Dragon

who have also seen this?) And the highlight of my stay in Montreal – the Jazz Festival, where the already lively streets were packed chocka with music lovers and revellers. The crêpe stalls were abundant, and the weather high. As well as much jazz in the streets of Montreal, I got to see a live Soul concert with Lulu and the Neville Brothers performing. Lulu had a dancer get up on the stage to dance with her but no complaints - I enjoyed some crêpes au chocolates, and again vowed to return one day to Montreal in some capacity or other. Many of these places I visited left an indelible mark on my psyche.

Quebec. Balthazaar. Train Station. The story here is that whilst I waited for my train at Montreal station I was standing next to a young man with a ticket for a seat next to mine. We got talking and it turned out that Balthazaar, a French teacher from Switzerland, was also going to stay in Quebec at L'Auberge de la Paix, 31 Couillard. And, coincidentally, we shared the same dormitory as well (rooms of 5 or 6 people in total). The buildings here are older, like Ottawa, traditional green-roofed buildings, presenting a very quaint town image. Quebec is possibly *the most* French city in Canada – more so than Montreal.

From the Château Fontainebleu on top of the hill, to the Plains of Abraham, down to the St Lawrence river, Quebec is French! As in Montreal you can find horses and carriages waiting to shuttle people around the city. You can find restaurants and bistros with authentic French menus and wine bars too. In the shop windows I saw various unusual items but remember one in particular, a stuffed polar bear, presumably from the Arctic. A bikers' parade rode through town one afternoon. Lord, I could stay at home in Helmsley, Yorkshire for that! Only these bikers were Harleys Angels or some such, so a point of interest there. Strolling round town, I saw a monument to King Louis XIV and the Notre Dame des Victoires cathedral.

Travelling with Balthazaar meant good company for a day or two, so we went to watch the changing of the guard at the Citadel. Here their regimental goat was on best behaviour as were the guards themselves and Balthazaar and I were able to take lots of photographs of the momentous occasion. They were wearing their red tunics and tall, black, furry hats which must have been very hot to wear in July.

Guess what? The Quebec Jazz Festival was in process! I had to go to one evening of live music. I have no idea who the artists were or what music they were playing, but it was a grand, spanking occasion. The performers were being recorded and on live Canadian television too, so I sat in the park (The Plains of Abraham – scene of an enormous siege and resistance in relatively recent military history) enjoying the sounds and the cool night breeze.

I was sad to leave Quebec, as this meant my travels were now over and my imminent return to Halifax meant an imminent return home to the UK. Anyway, I caught the train at 22:07 Friday, 8th July, and arrived in Halifax 16:20 the next day, after a long, overnight 18 hour train ride. In Halifax I stayed at the Youth Hostel, as Fenwick were adamant about no takers without a residence contract. In this hostel I met Jerome, a school teacher from the remote Northern Territories. As I was leaving the next day I gave him half a packet of Swedish meatballs for dinner and in return we had a conversation about UK schooling and Science Fiction writing, especially that by Tad Williams. So my stay in the hostel meant Halifax from a new perspective. I called Ruth and Paul to arrange transport to the airport, and simultaneously heard on the News that there had been the 7th July London bombings. What exactly was I flying back to? Ruth and Paul put me up for a night and then bade me farewell at Halifax airport on the afternoon of Sunday, July 10th 2005. I arrived in London in the early hours of Monday, July 11th (08:25am) and phoned my brother Chris for directions to cross London with all my baggage. I did so, and met him at his local tube station, presenting him with two bottles of Canadian beverage....Canadian Rye, and Canadian Ice Wine. I spent several days in London before returning home to Yorkshire and back with family.

The Green Dragon

This concluded my Canadian exchange year.

Chapter Seven
Marathon

So it all began on a school sports day back in 1986. This chapter details my athletic record, beginning with a Primary school 50 yard dash and culminating in a 26.2 miler – the Paris Marathon. The fact that there were about twenty years in between can also be accounted for. The fact that it was in response to my brother Chris's running the New York marathon of 2000 is also to be understood.

In a nutshell, I always enjoyed running when I was a kid. That 50 yard dash saw me gaining my first ever accolade for sport – a yellow ribbon pinned to my t-shirt for coming second. I was really proud of this yellow ribbon. James Halkon won the race, and Barry Foots followed closely home in third.

At this point the full-lap race seemed a rare and mysterious event indeed. I didn't enjoy distance running until my final year at Terrington, five years later, when I won the 400m and 800m, and came second to Marcus Smith in the 3.5 mile cross country. The school magazine published my photo in that race, though, so I was chuffed with that turn of events.

At Terrington we had a regular weekly school run on a Thurday afternoon with Tim Chapman, Martin Wright, Tim Anderson, Ken Starks, and John Hamer supervising. I always looked forwards to improving my time each week and seeing whom I could beat. Will Machin, David O'Gram, Bonner Earle and Marcus Smith were amongst the best distance runners at Terrington in my time. I was always on the school team, though, when we were competing.

I left Terrington with my head held high, knowing that I could be good at something, and even beat others at the same time. I went on to Durham School aged 13 and in my first year, my running got me noticed. I did well in the junior Kingston and Swainston runs, and won some races at sports day – again 800m and

The Green Dragon

1500m. These results repeated themselves over the next three years, with times gradually getting faster, distances increasing and competitition more taxing. I gained my house and school colours for athletics, cross-country, and music over the five year period at Durham.

William Bishop beat me in the Junior Swainston and then again in the Senior Dunelmian (10 miles) a year later. I came 2nd three times; once to Edwin James – a nationals standard runner. William Bishop lost a trainer halfway round but never stopped. He won the race and was on crutches for weeks afterwards! The other significant race was the notoriously hilly Kingston. I won the Intermediate and Senior races at least once each, in different years, and we had Steve Cram come to talk to us at an Athletics Society dinner one year. I gave a humble captain's speech at the event. At my peak I had earned 4th place in a Durham City race, and was on the Durham County squad. I used to get a big head about my school trophies, which peeved some people.

At this time I was vaguely aware of the World and European Championships, Olympics, and Commonwealth Games, having witnessed the 1997 world cross-country championships in Durham, but it all seemed so far away, as though I was not on the same planet. These were a light year away from schoolboy athletics and although I had been inspired by the 1992 Barcelona Olympics on telly as well, I never twigged on to them. Anyway, in truth, my fastest 800m time was merely 2mins 12secs so I shouldn't have even entertained the idea. I was a mile off! When I left school I fancied that I could win Olympic Gold at some event or other but my delusion was grand and got me into a lot of bother one way or the other. I tried my hand at taekwondo for a while, but only got to green tag level. I left school shortly after this and struggled to locate a new dojo to learn from when I lived with my parents. But this went pear-shaped.

For the next several years I lost all interest in keeping fit, running, and athletics. It was only in 2001 after a spell in hospital that I joined Pickering Running Club with the intention of completing the Great North Run 2002. Leading up to this event I ran every week with the club, whilst living in Malton, North Yorkshire. We attended many events, and I ran the following 10km road races in under an hour: Scarborough 2002, Walkington 2002, and Kirbymoorside 2002. When the time came to run the Great North Run I had just started University at Hull, but still ran from the Pickering club bus. I wore a t-shirt for Leukaemia research and raised over £500 that time. I ran the race slowly in 2hrs 12 mins, but was really proud to have completed it at all. Back to Hull the next day and on with a new schedule.

Ever since I was 18, I had wanted to run the London marathon, and knew that I had what it would take to do so. However, over those years I applied three times and got turned down each time for one reason or another. My eldest brother Chris had flown to New York, USA, in November 2000 and ran their marathon in 3hrs 37mins. He showed us all his pictures very proudly back home when he came back. At that time he had been living and working in London for many years, making his way in the big world. I was impressed! I wanted to do the same, but in a different way.

As it transpired, it took me six years to build up fitness for the Paris marathon of April 2006, although, technically, I committed to a 15 month training plan which began whilst I was abroad in Canada. I entered for the Halifax 10km (Nova Scotia), May 2005, and ran in the pouring rain, coming home in about an hour. There was also a full distance marathon underway that day and to see them setting off to the tune of 'Eye of the Tiger' really inspired me. I definitely wanted to run a marathon from then on.

Flying back to England was an unwelcome event in my life, but the exchange year had elapsed so I came home to finish off at Hull. Incidentally, one in-flight movie I saw was about a 14 year old boy called Ralph who fictitiously won the Boston marathon, USA. This also inspired me.

In Hull I joined the Athletics club and we ran various 10km road races and half marathons, 2005-06, prior to my big race, including Bridlington – November 2005 (1hr 46mins), and Bath – March 2006 (1hr 30mins). Additionally, I covered 12-15 miles regularly on a Sunday training route over the months. I had a training partner called Ben Dudgeon who also ran a marathon (London 2006). He was a drama student, played saxophone, and drove a Mini Cooper. Other runs I completed were the following 10km – Elloughton 2005 (Uncle Frank, Mum and Dad came to witness this), Harrogate 2005, Broughton 2005 plus training routes of the same distance on the streets of Hull.

I attempted to train with the Harriers of Hull Costello Stadium. I was outclassed instantly, but once joined them for a session on the Westwood Pastures of Beverley where I ran barefoot for an hour and a half in the muddy grass. One afternoon a week I swam a mile in an hour at the Beverley Road baths. Two mornings a week I played competitive squash and often won my games in the sports centre. On a Monday evening I did circuit training in the main hall with other athletes and keep-fit students. I had been involved with games of tennis, badminton, juggling and trampolining during my time at Hull.

Rather than catch a bus I preferred to walk to and from town to the shops. It was only a half hour walk, and it helped keep my weight down at the time. I was ten and a half stone at my peak of fitness and getting slimmer by the day. Alfie, a gym instructor, kept monitoring me and getting concerned about this lack of body fat. Jo Teehan was also a gym instructor but didn't like me much so I never got to train with Jo. I had a full leg massage every fortnight leading up to the marathon. This helped relieve muscular tension. Also, I practised yoga, meditation and deep breathing exercises at home to remain balanced. I felt really powerful when fit.

My diet was controlled to the extent of having a food chart on my kitchen cupboard. Every time I ate something I would note how much protein, carbohydrate, sugar, fibre, fat or salt was in that food product. It got ridiculous after a while as I could hardly eat anything without finding fault somehow. The fitter I was, the less sleep I needed. Morning wakeups were anywhere between 5am-7am, 2005-2006. I had a part time job at a Ramada Jarvis hotel as bar staff/waiter. This required transport and flexible hours. I preferred to give my time to marathon training, though, so left the job after some months.

By the time April 2006 arrived I was fit and ready to run, and had raised the prerequisite £1000 for Get Kids Going, who organised sports equipment for kids with special needs. I felt champion! The National Express coach took me to London, there I met up with brother Chris and sister-in-law Emma before catching the midnight bus from London Victoria to Paris via a Dover-Calais ferry in the early hours. I practised yoga on the open deck to get some fresh air but could hardly sleep a wink on the bus for listening to MP3s all night.

In Paris I visited the Sacre Coeur, Notre Dame, Arc de Triomphe, Champs Elysées, and Paris Conservatoire of Music. I was there in spirit alright as well as body. I met Chris and Emma for lunch in a Paris restaurant the day before the race. I was lost for words, though. They had very kindly spared the time to come and support my run. I got to my hotel room for an early night only to discover my room mate yelling at me for wanting to get up at 5am on race day. I did anyway, and practised my stretches, yoga and breathing and even said a prayer to the Good Lord himself for a good run ahead. All my kit was prepared to put straight on in the morning.

I was on my own now, and at the start line had bagged up tracksuit and assorted items. I peed into an empty bottle and then the claxon sounded. Wherever we ran that day it was a pleasure, a hard but gratifying pleasure. They had many banana pitstops and assorted fruit and drinks along the way. I only stopped once for a pee but everyone probably saw this as I pulled over by a tree.

The weather was fair and there was no rain or hard wind to contend with. I looked out for other runners wearing the same charity t-shirt as myself. Because I had written my name on my t-shirt an occasional cheer of support would be offered. I never saw Chris and Emma, nor they me, until the end of the race. There were plenty of pictures though, for proof. We ran down the Champs Elysées across to Parc de l'Est, then back west to Bois de Boulogne before sailing home in 3hrs 25mins. I had done it – I beat Chris's New York time by ten minutes!

During the wind down all runners were offered a medal, bananas, water, and a space blanket to keep them warm. Some went for a massage, but queues were long so I got straight off to meet Chris and Emma again. Sure enough, there they were waiting at the 'K' stand with big grins on their faces. We were chilling out on the lawn when a gorilla walked past – someone had run the course in a gorilla costume!

So that was a dream come true – I had run a marathon. At Hull University, one of my lecturers – Steve Braund – who was himself a trained triathlete, offered congratulations and inspired me to want to try a triathlon.

Back home, I must have inspired my friends David Goodwin and Sam Belsom to run because David was in for the Great North Run, October 2006, (and I was too, but circumstances prevented my participation), and Sam went on to run the Kirbymoorside 10km road race, and the Castle Howard 10km run some time later.

The last time I ran an official road event was the Beverley 10km of May, 2007. I had had time out in hospital so was glad just to get round the course and my dad had driven especially to watch the occasion. I enjoyed my running days. Athletics was good for me. I was born 1978, and the first Olympics in my life were: Moscow 1980 with Seb Coe going for 1500m Gold, Steve Cram in hot pursuit. 1984 Los Angeles, 1988 Seoul (Steve Redgrave's first Gold), 1992 Barcelona (Linford Christie's World's Fastest Man), 1996 Atlanta (Michael Johnson's 12-year-standing 100m Olympic/World record made here), 2000 Sydney, 2004 Athens (Steve Redgrave's 5th/Matthew Pinsent's 4th), 2008 Beijing (Usain Bolt's World Records 100m, 200m, Jamaican Relay Team), to London 2012. For some there can be nothing other!

**Chapter Eight
Sectioned Again**

A July afternoon 2006. Sun shining, no wind. Perfect summer time.

There I was, washing the dishes, wondering what chores would be next on the list, when out of the blue, all of a sudden Dad appeared at the back door with two social workers, and Mum at the front door with two doctors.

With a split second decision to make, I scrambled upstairs to put on my shoes and hat, and I just knew that I had to get out of this untimely, unwelcome predicament. So with the words, "I have no time for you freaks, you aliens……you are not f***ing welcome in my life – excuse me please!" I vacated the premises.

My first manoeuvre was simply to walk up the street to the Howl woods. Whereby I figured to take a sharp diversion into the top fields. There I meditated calmly, took some deep breaths and stretched my entire physique using standard technique and yoga, following which I walked across the field to be chased by a gipsy's dog – who quickly made good friends with me. From here I walked round the back of Nawton County Primary School on to the playing fields where a local cricket match was being played. As I sat there at the pavilion for fifteen minutes I witnessed sixes and fours being scored a 'dozen at a time'. Also, Mark Rymer was spectating, so I said "Hello" to him after all those years without seeing him.

Then, round about that time I got to figuring that I should not go back home but, rather, should get to other places. But where to go? York? (Jonny's place), Bradford? (Jonty's place), or London? (Chris and Emma's place), Hull? (friends from university), or even somewhere completely different? I made a conscious decision – run to York there and then and tell my brother that we should form a band.

The Green Dragon

Prior to setting out, from Beadlam, I went to the field at the top of our street, sat in the branches of a big, fat tree and urinated onto the sheep passing below me in the field, following which, the farmer stormed across the field to clear me off. I pulled a moony, raised my middle finger, and off I trotted – down the fields through Wombleton, across the aerodrome, then to Nunnington – up the farm track to Caulkley's bank top and down the other side to Hovingham (by which point it was now nightfall and the temperature cooling rapidly. I was wearing my magic Pearl Izumi training shoes, Patrick tracksuit pants, pink Teddy Smith t-shirt and a turquoise baseball cap. Drinkers at the Worsley Arms no doubt speculated as I ran past them in the cool evening). Up the Hovingham hill and towards Terrington. In between these two spots I got scared, running in the pitch black dark woods so began to shout really loudly, "I need to win!!" which gave me sufficient reassurance to continue on my journey.

When I got to Terrington bank top I stopped to admire the view for five minutes and to catch my breath. I was half way – I had jogged approximately twelve miles already! Then on to Sheriff Hutton, but just before the incline leading up to the village a police van had cottoned on to me, as somebody must have telephoned when they heard the shouting. The officer requested that I stop but I made no actual compliance with this.

In Sheriff Hutton a second officer had already been summoned in a van to cut me off. However, as the vans interacted and the officers demanded, I sneaked through the small gap in between the van bonnet and a building to discover an officer and police dog chasing me on foot. He was brandishing a truncheon and screaming, "Kill him, Barney!" (to the dog), so my only means of evasion now were impromptu and instinctive – I ran fast through a gap in the hedge into the playing field area.

Neither Barney the German Shepherd nor the Officers knew to follow me here – so the chase came to a temporary stand still. Now I undertook some fence climbing and "à la Boyz in the Hood" found myself jumping through people's back gardens in the dead of night. Eventually I came to open hay fields and ran again.

Whilst navigating by moonlight I heard a helicopter coming in my direction with search-light glaring. So I simply jumped across the road to the other side and hid in a hedge-row for some time. Once in a while I would look up to discover the searchlight scouring the fields, outhouses and hedge-rows, so I made no move.

Then inspiration struck – run in the opposite direction – further away. So off I darted to a local forest and skirted the edge by moonlight. Fortunately there was no rain and no real wind, just a calm summer's night. All the while I watched the chopper's searchlight shining.

Then I guessed that a police trap might be in store if I were to carry on to York, so I doubled back, walked through Bulmer and by first light reached the A64. Here I found some milk to drink at the Jinnah restaurant for breakfast, and walked cross-country all day through fields, woods and streams until at night-time I scrambled over a tall fence behind McDonald's, tumbling into the garden shrubs nearly causing myself an injury, and walked along the banks of the River Ouse to Jonny's place arriving by about eleven p.m.

Jonny gave me food to eat, a bath to wash myself, ointment for my scratches, a comfy bed for the night, and £10 for my troubles. First thing in the morning I walked to York station and caught a Virgin train to Leeds. The train was so busy that the conductor never asked me for a ticket so I travelled for free.

Here I was to decide – Bradford? Or other? I chose other, deciding to get away from it all – destination determined to be The Pennine Way. So from Leeds there were two options – either a) I walk along the Leeds-Liverpool canal towpath and join the Pennine Way at Gargrave, or b) catch the train to Ilkley and walk from there.

As it happens I caught the train to Ilkley, and again no conductor appeared to ask for tickets, so free travel again. Hooray, hoorah!

Once at Ilkley, I mooched around the shops for an hour, then set off on foot once again by the roadside to Skipton. The weather was sunny but with a cool wind. I was now in possession of a long-sleeved sweatshirt jumper which helped keep me warm.

On the way, the footpath went up a long farm-track to a cattle farm and through a field of bullocks. The entire herd of bullocks began to follow me as I walked, so the farmer pulled over in his tractor raging "Where the f*** do you think you are going to?" including some additional gestures and expletives, of course. I told him simply, "I'm going to Skipton". This satisfied the farmer, although clearly perplexed by his cattle following a complete stranger – no doubt worrying that I would walk them right the way to Skipton market?! My theory to this day is that my jumper was a black and white Adidas top, so the black and white cattle could identify with me.

Once in Skipton, following a long six-mile roadside walk, I moved to the sheltered woodlands on suspicion that undercover officers were on to me again. I saw people talking through oral-intercoms in town. Here at Skipton there was a Tourist Information Centre which gave a free map of the Pennine Way and I called at a local bar for a glass of water and a sandwich (apart from which wild woodland raspberries were all I ate, and cow-byre water to drink). I gorged myself on wild berries. Then I continued to walk along the roadside until I arrived at Gargrave. Here the canal (Leeds-Liverpool) intersects with the Pennine Way. So finally I had arrived at destination point A.

The Pennine Way: Location Gargrave.

The first sign-post popped up so I gladly followed it, walking along the canal-side. A lock-keeper wished me well on my journey and continued to keep the lock in fully functional order.

I walked around the narrow roadway to find where the hillside track was due to commence.

A mile and a half walk on the road and then field/woodland. Over a fence I saw a blue zipper-bag dumped in the woods, but for two reasons I did not climb the fence to unzip the bag. Reason number one – the spirits of the forest all warded me away from the baggage, and reason number two – a car full of 'likely' youths had just passed by the scene – so I felt unnerved and carried on my way.

At the top of the first hill I looked round, and down at the bottom – en route – was a field full of cattle and further on the track two workmen with chainsaws and mallets. By now with no food to eat, I began to feel wary and paranoid. So my mental health had begun to suffer already. Incidentally – the first night had been without sleep…I was moving all night long. The second night, Jonny had given me a place to stay over, so now I was in possession of £10. What to do with this?

Having layed down paranoically trying to determine whether the workmen would try to decapitate me with their chainsaw, I spent half an hour deep in thought on that hill top on The Pennine Way.

Determining to venture forth, I picked myself up and walked on my merry way on the path. As I walked past the workmen, they simply proceeded to go about their craft, continuing to erect a new fence, building whatever it was that they were building. Much to my gratification I was not decapitated and I got to carry on along the Pennine Way that afternoon.

All evening I continued walking – past a "highest point monolith". The views were tremendous. Outstanding Yorkshire Dales scenery unfolded before my eyes all around. All that I knew now was that I was going North to Scotland, or The Lake District. As I walked on, I felt privileged to be a Yorkshireman walking in God's country. The whole colour scheme appealed to my aesthetic side. Fields, streams, forests, clouds in the sky,

The Green Dragon

birds in the air, sheep in the fields. Not a soul in sight except for me out in the blissful countryside open air.

On this day I kept on walking and walking until I arrived at Malham, by dusk. With £10 in my pocket there was nowhere to stay, but the local Inn made me a hot lemon drink and sent me on my merry way (The Buck Inn). Not knowing exactly where to spend the night I figured on walking up the hill to the famous Malham Tarn itself, some three miles up the road up an exceedingly steep hill and all in the dark. Cloud cover meant that there was precious little moonlight to lighten my path on this occasion, and the night was cold and windy with gathering precipitation the higher up I climbed.

Up the hill, and up higher and higher until finally I reached a clear, flat area with roads to walk along on. Walking past a field of snoring, sleeping cows, and through the quiet stillness of that night I carried on.

Eventually I reached a woodland area and the Tarn itself. Although this night was spent on top of an overlooking hill within a cairn 'windshelter' – my only concerns before dropping off to sleep were with any local gryphons, lions, cougars, or moorland panthers/monsters which might eat me up over an open grave.

Fortunately, my luck was in – I woke up the next morning at first light fully intact and bemused by the entire proceedings. So, down the hill to Malham Tarn itself where I splashed my face with water and paddled out up to my knees before marching on.

Unbeknown to me then, just around the corner was a Research Field Study Centre. As it happens they had left their kitchen and bathroom windows wide open – not expecting any unrequested company, no doubt. So at a distance I unlaced my shoes and emptied my pockets of everything. Then I proceeded to tip-toe back to the building with the intention of exploration and food acquisition.

At first I climbed in through the bathroom window and walked into the main hallway only to discover a rather deterring laser 'burglar' alarm in view ready to sound the alarm if an intruder like me were to walk in. So, consequently I returned out of the bathroom window and relocated to the kitchen window for re-entry.

A gauze attached by Velcro needed to be unfastened at first, and so this took some time at 5:30 a.m. so as not to wake anybody up. Inside the kitchen there was fruit, cereal, and a freezer full of potato-chips and other assorted vegetables. I took an orange, an apple, and a bag of croquet potatoes with me, leaving a note reading, "Thankyou, Malham!" Back out of the window, around the far side of the building a lounge window was wide open, so I reached in and took a bottle of wine with me for the day ahead. A full-bodied Red at that! Very delicious – yes, thankyou Malham indeed.

Back on the trail, more walking, miles and miles, with my nice Skipton TIC map for directions and wine with croquet potatoes for sustenance. Great stuff!

Finally it happened – I felt tired after miles of gorgeous and beautiful scenery, hills, dales and vales – there was the sudden need to sleep again, drunk on wine and frozen potato. So, I lay down and slept.

After however long (wearing no watch), I woke up again and picked up from the hillside, seeing the mountain 'Pen-y-Ghent' right in front of me. Still a sunny yet cool day, an unusual encounter occurred here as I took the wrong turn. Rather than walking a mile down the road to the proper track, I ventured cross-country (by mistake) and stumbled through the heather and bracken. A grouse/pheasant-hunter approached me with his dog and rifle.

"Where are you going?" he demanded. "Steer clear of this moorland – you are scaring the grouse!"

The Green Dragon

He seemed upset and aggressive so I did not wish to upset him any further. I offered him some wine and potatoes. "No, thanks", he responded, then proceeded to advise me how to climb Pen-y-Ghent. "Follow the wall right round and then you will get to the track".

"Thankyou very much, sir" I answered, feeling obliged.

Instead of heeding his advice, I climbed straight up the side of Pen-y-Ghent like a mountain goat. I am certain that he took some shots at me with his rifle to scare me. The sounds were like those of rifle fire and ricocheting bullets!

Fortunately again, I arrived at the top of the mountain unharmed, still carrying the bottle of red wine and bag of potato chips. At the top I finished drinking the wine and placed the bottle on the marker-stone. Quite a number of other people also were there at the top (but they had walked up the proper route)...thankfully! Glad to see human company once again.

I took no rest and proceeded to walk down the path to pursue my destiny. Only (unbeknown to me then) I was going back the exact way I had just come from. Two miles on I was back to the road that I had originally left. What to do? Consult the map and march straight back again. What a carry on!

Back at the top of Pen-y-Ghent I passed several other hikers en route and continued, after suffering the double climb (by my own failing judgement), down the far side to the village of Horton in Ribblesdale. There I stopped at the village pub for lots of _water_ to drink.

From here I walked on, but lost The Pennine Way route somehow, so ended up willy-nilly in the Yorkshire Dales for hours on end. Beautiful as the scenery all was presented, I had no fucking clue as to where exactly I was then. But on I walked.

All I remember here is that there was a long open exposed hilltop, and the only company I had was some geographical surveyor buzzing overhead in a helicopter. Apart from this, I was the only human being for miles around. That is literally, miles and miles and miles. Remote, tranquil, peaceful – you name it!

Somewhere in between here and Thwaite, the route went through a field full of fully-grown bullocks. They seemed particularly frisky in their behaviour so I did not wish to fancy my chances with them. Running faster would have been an option – that is if I was up to running at all. I observed a route around the top of the field, so opted for that. Only, before I set off I sat for twenty minutes chatting to the beasts about irony…would you believe, they all gathered round the field wall where I was seated and listened like school children. I even gave the bullocks individual names but can no longer recall what they were. They appeared an intelligent and captive audience so my words were no doubt appreciated!

Gradually, day turned into night and I found myself being bleated at by sheep – loudly, very loudly. Moving down the hillside I saw an outdoor bonfire and heard a group of people celebrating something. No doubt a summer vacation or suchlike. So I sat speculating, watching from a hillside at a distance, until it dawned on me that some of the people who had seen me earlier, and were concerning themselves with my business on the hillside.

As men with flashlights came up the hill I crossed many gates until finally I found a peaceful alcove to spend the night – in the open by a streamside. The stream trickled through the cold night. Although the night's sleep was rough/intermittent, at first light I got back on the road, walking towards Hawes. I found that I had got seven miles off the Pennine Way overnight by travelling willy-nilly. Bad thing – so I followed the road right into Hawes village.

There at an inn, I found 20p, so now my capital had risen by 2%. Fantastic! Also, a chance to rest my feet. Today's mission decided…to arrive at Thwaite for lunchtime and put my feet up

The Green Dragon

for some time. Sure enough, though dairy farming seemed prevalent in Hawes, with its dairy/cheese/milk factory, I carried on to Thwaite. On the way to Thwaite, another mountainous high point unfolded before me. There were no other people in sight or sound, so I lay down to rest by the cairn. I slept – for ages. Must have been really hungry by now. Tired, lost, cold, hungry and thirsty.

On awakening, I saw a group of hikers fast approaching. One, two, three, four young men with rucksacks coming towards me. So quickly I stood up in the by now searing sunlight (midday July sunshine) and got a move on before they could catch me up.

But they were walking quickly and did catch me up, offering water to drink. I did not like that they stopped for a smoke so continued at a rapid pace down the track to Thwaite. There an inn-keeper gave me a jug of water with ice and lemon to drink.

Unfortunately the tender demanded £1 just for a jug of water plus ice and lemon which I could not believe. I refused to pay the £1 charge and drank the water. The tender at this point flew into a rage and almost smashed the glass over my head. Something within the man prevented this from occurring – thankyou, God! Here I sat in their beer garden but was requested to leave the premises owing to the lack of payment.

I walked round the corner to the stream. Here I took off my shoes and socks and, sitting down on a rock, dipped my blistered feet into the cool running water and washed my footwear as well.

After 20 minutes of this soothing there were voices coming from the village green so I hobbled over to join the four young men who had met me on the trail earlier in the day. They asked me a few questions and determined from my responses that I needed food. The guy named Simon bought me a bacon and sausage sandwich with a drink. Also, he gave me Kendal mint cake, spare socks and a space blanket to keep warm at night. Thankyou very much, kind sir - -I really appreciated this act very much.

The four chaps suggested I walk with them on the trail and set off once again. So there they were (four guys), and there I was, heading for Keld with only a bottle for water and a belly full of food now. Good vittles! I kept up walking for a while – only for the group to sit down suddenly and tell me to eat noodles. They cooked me noodles and gave me more drink. As I approached them there was a change of heart. They decided jointly that I needed help so went to call for a doctor. One of the group returned to Thwaite to call a doctor for me. "Rats!" I thought. So I charged off on my own over the hills, leaving this group of four behind.

Incidentally, a fully grown bull had smelt the noodles cooking and heard the noise so came to inspect us at closer quarters. Fortunately, the bull retreated into the field and made no further inspection of us in any manner.

I remember knocking on a young lady's hillside home door to request water. Her dog (a little terrier) attacked me with maximum intent, but she happily gave me some fresh water. Then finally I walked down a seriously steep hill to the roadside where I walked on again.

Feeling paranoid, I headed past a river full of men, women and children paddling, ducking and diving. I made into a field and sat on the rocks by the stream, eating the Kendal mint cake which had been given me earlier by the four hikers.

Then suddenly a Police car pulled up in the gateway and there was no escape as a sheer cliff prevented a stream crossing and the only gateway was there. So I walked over to them.

On being questioned I had given my name as Steven Morris, and my destination as The Lake District. They arrested me gently. No brute force. I was feeling tired, confused, perplexed, and was no doubt delirious, too.

The Officers (one middle-aged male, one middle-aged female) chatted to me the whole journey. They nearly took me to

The Green Dragon

Catterick Army Garrison to drop me off there. But they drove me to Northallerton Police Station. There I spent the night in the cells. Some Psychiatrist came to question me, but I was more interested in exercising and pulling headstands on the mattress than talking to anybody.

So there we have it. Caught in Keld! Driven to Northallerton Police Station, and then transferred to St Luke's Hospital, Middlesbrough, in the early hours of a summer's morning.

There my first impressions were of a tiny nurse who I am sure was heavily into dirty pornography. I yelled 'You're all crazy' and 'Bastardos!' as they pinned me down and injected me with Haloperidol and Lorazepam in my buttocks. I spat in someone's face and punched the manager on the nose, causing a nose bleed; get in there, fella!

The nurse subsequently gave me a 500 piece jigsaw of a kitten – presumably to calm me down - and for some reason I accepted the challenge and completed it within a week. That was the beginning of a new hobby for me. I named the kitten 'Aslan', then did another 500 piece puzzle of a rabbit, 'Cracker', then a 1000-piece Egyptian pyramid puzzle. Dad visited and took a photo of this when completed – actually only 999 pieces available! Where did the missing piece go?

Then I did a 500-piece puzzle of a sail boat, helped by the nurses. Then a 300-piece jigsaw of field mice. I was all jigsawed out by this time. I wanted to have sex with a nurse. She told me to masturbate. The bastards condemned me for being in shape. When Steve Irwin got killed by a stingray I cried. When Kenenisa Bekele won the 10,000m race I yelled support at the TV. When the proms were on I listened and talked about different instruments. We talked about dogs – whippets. I carried a soft toy dog called Pépé with me at all times, whom I considered to be my pet and lucky mascot. One nurse thought it strange and tried to insinuate to the Doctor about my mental health because of this.

My Doctor told me of his own experience when I told him I felt outstanding. What would he know about running marathons? Whilst he was getting paid £150,000 a year I was obliged to be signing on benefits once again. Disaster movie or what. Another Doctor came to visit to talk about Scarborough. He had me out in the yard doing triple jump, basketball and bought me a can of shandy. One staff nurse tried to educate me about the racing pages, how to interpret the horses. I talked to him about the Olympics. The Games had me gripped at that time, as I was then 'marathon-fit'. Suffering by attrition on the wards my fitness gradually waned. All my life was suddenly slipping through my fingertips as I lay locked in the ward.

I did enjoy the Therapy sessions doing art and cooking and making music and walking round the grounds breathing deeply. I wanted to marry one student nurse. Maybe could have asked her. She was very beautiful as well. I imagined her riding my cock like a jockey on a stallion.

I made bread and shared it round with everyone. Having Christian allusions at the time, I looked a bit like Jesus with long hair and a goatee beard. The chaplain – Paul Walker – came to see me, as did Mike, the other chaplain, still there since 2001. I did a mosaic of a Gryffon in therapy which I ended up giving to Chris and Emma for their then London home.

One girl had a baby there and didn't seem to notice very much. Debby gave me a kiss. Janet played keyboard – Seal's 'Kiss from a rose'. Alex turned up one day in Therapy.

Another staff nurse seemed alright to me – he talked with me sometimes humanely and told me about a bonfire he had attended with his friends whilst camping. But in the Doctor's meetings it was him writing the notes, though.

Someone called Dean Graeme was there – previously a band member, guitarist and singer from Seachimp. We got on well briefly, and played Scrabble once, inventing ridiculous words all

The Green Dragon

the while, such as 'Deansyaloop'. He sang and played guitar. Said he thought he was Jesus. He told me his band had split up, but I could use the name Seachimp for my story if I wanted – take it or leave it he said! I used the name in my first book Plan 103f.

A female nurse was fit, slim and wanted my babies. She would have gone with me if I had asked. Reluctantly administering medicine to my fit body, the path of destruction was being laid.

Too much food and not enough exercise. One morning around 3am I wanted to go for a jog so got my tracksuit on, stretched and prepared mentally, then stepped out of my room to go. Two staff members prevented me from going. I called them 'incompetent peckers'. They called back-up and flattened me once again in my room and injected me with more medicine. I had had enough by this point.

Where did the love go? Let the good times roll, oh baby, let the good times roll. At one point, as the nurses prepared to inject me, I threw a television through the window in disgust. The whole set-up cried of heart attacks and death. Stinking squalor.

They ended up sending me back to Cross Lane, Scarborough. I had attempted previously to learn guitar and harmonica whilst there. Also, I walked around pretending to be blind with my eyes shut, stripped naked, and was escorted back to my room to put on clothes. I took ice baths to maintain my leg muscles – fat lot of good my marathon training ended up doing for me. Banned from life, banned from my own brilliant reality.

They ignored my marathon, my pure blood and filled me with horrors, ignominy, toxins and petty health and safety policy. Not even a handstand permitted. Just sit, eat, watch telly, and don't breathe too much lest you distract the smokers. Fucking jokers.

December 2006 on the news – Alexander Litvinyenko, Russian KGB agent, was 'silenced', and Saddam Hussein, Iraqi President, was hanged.

One person whom I met in hospital was Paul Wilson. We both played viola, and he had been to the Royal College of Music in London some time earlier. He also played piano and guitar very well. We had a bit of a jam one afternoon and that seemed to impress a nurse very much at the time. Paul was brought up in Malton, where I visited him once or twice after hospital. He also lived in York for a while, where I had hoped to live myself. That didn't happen – nevermind. In town one day I bought tennis wristbands with Wilson written on them to mark the friendship, and later when I visited Paul I sneaked him some French Red Wine and some Fosters to drink! A bit risky as alcohol was banned on the wards. Paul went on to write symphonies for the Teeside County Orchestra, and he lives in Middlesbrough today.

In Scarborough I was attracted to a certain female nurse. However, she was equally deceitful, suggestively bending over furniture when we were alone in the living room, and putting on the film 'Hideously Kinky' – again when it was just the two of us. The only problem was they all posed as friends, but the truth was far removed from a friendship. Like anybody who sits in authority or judgement – your subjects are all OK, so long as they go along with what you are telling them. Everything is just fine until somebody knows better and beats them at their own game. In that case – bloody murder, literally physically, mentally, and emotionally assaulted by the bastards every time. Every time! That's my experience of the NHS mental health system anyway. I did know better, I was achieving more, I was highly athletic, smart, hardworking and I had started to win in life. All I prayed for was victory. But I was locked up and stuffed full of toxins and left to rot in the corner. Behaved, did I? Try being roped, gagged, bound and branded.

My eldest brother Chris got engaged during this time. The lovely Emma Maurice had agreed to marry him in the South of France, both having lived and worked in London for over a decade. I prepared a 1000 piece art puzzle by Jim Zuckerman for their Christmas present 2006. Very fine. Occupational Therapy taught me some basic blues on guitar. I got on fine with them at Therapy, and met Nick Marshall for the first time in Therapy where I prepared collages and various pictures. Nick eventually moved to work in York with Credit Union but we did bump into each other several times later over the years. I often read poetry and listened to NLP discs by the Australian author/cartoonist Andrew Matthews.

One evening I was playing snakes and ladders with a staff nurse and I decided that if I won with my lucky boot I would run away. I won. So I went to get my jacket and hat, asked to get some fresh air and promptly climbed the fence. I went to York by train, but Jonny was out, so I went on to Leeds and Bradford. Jonty was out, so I went to JJB sports shop in Bradford and bought a BMX with a new store card – USC Duet. I rode about Bradford town for a while, then caught the train back to York where I stayed by the river Ouse pulling stunts all night, cycling round town and up to the Racecourse. I tried to sleep rough on the benches and it turns out that Jonny and Jonty had seen a 'strange and mysterious cyclist' on the way home from a night out. They didn't know it was me until later on when I told them. I also climbed Clifford's Tower embankment with some teens on sledges, and I rode down on my BMX, promptly causing some scrapes and cuts as I fell. The next day I left my bike with Jonny and caught the train back to Scarborough and walked back to hospital.

In order to rehydrate I had lots of water to drink, then tried to run away again – I really hadn't intended to be there. I was stopped one night and escorted back onto the ward and asked how I got out? The bathroom window had been unlocked and I feigned having a bath. Another time I went to the 'Scholars' bar for a drink then called a taxi to take me to Teeside airport at 1am. I tried to buy a ticket to Amsterdam first thing in the morning where I had been supposed to run the marathon in October 2006, but the airport police stopped me, probably disbelieving my story, and my credit card was frozen, anyway. I walked into

Darlington town early that morning where I was totally stuck – no money, cold, exhausted, and lost, and made a reverse-charge call to my brother Chris but no ticket was possible so I ended up handing myself in at Darlington Police station for evading my Mental Health Section.

They held me for questioning then drove me handcuffed to Sutton Bank Top. A second police van was there and I was handed over uncuffed and bundled into the back of the van. I felt sick on the way to Scarborough as they drove quickly to Cross Lane Hospital. There I was looked after under close observation for the rest of the section time. A red-headed nurse removed my shoes and socks whilst I lay on my bed. I felt like a prize plonker by now.

One guy continued to laugh a lot and talked in depth about girls and his music. Martin was my next door neighbour and frequently made allusions to rap music, breaking into many a verse in his own right. I learnt beginner's Spanish and Russian whilst there. In physio they took care of things and we played table tennis and used the gym. On the ward I played guitar, organ, and harmonica often in my room. Physio staff took some of us swimming on a Friday afternoon. Compared to my previous regime I found it almost impossible to adjust. That was the end of my innocence as far as I'm concerned.

Round about January 2007 I had been offered some housing forms for an independent flat on Sussex Street for two years. The flats were run by Rethink/Yorkshire Coast Homes and I would be interviewed soon on condition of moving into 2 Trafalgar Square until a place became available in the flats.

Of course, I snapped up the opportunity to have my 'own place' to live, and filled in the form with my mum providing a detailed reference. February – May 2007 I lived in a bedsit room in Trafalgar Square as a supported respite. In truth, I actually enjoyed my time here, resting, reading, playing badminton, tennis, chatting, cooking, group walks and other activities offered too. One of my nurses actually made sure that when I moved to Sussex Court I was given a 'furnishings grant' to buy all mod cons with, including sofa and armchair. They awarded me over £600 for all the following: wardrobe, 2 chests of drawers, writing bureau, telephone, sofa, armchair, corner cabinet, kitchen utensils, kettle, toaster, and sandwich maker, plus other items too. I was blessed! Fortunately somebody was starting to appear as my Social worker at this time and seemed to understand where I was coming from. He got me referred to Dr Mogyorosy (Consultant Psychiatrist) and we seemed to get on just fine. No worries about female deceit, lies or gender manipulation at this point in time.

I got moved into Sussex Court and was given my keys by about May 20th, 2007; then signed the two-year contract gladly. Thanks to the following Rethink staff I had a relatively 'free' two years at that address, enjoying saving money, writing, making music and personal space as well. I had my own bathroom, kitchen, bedroom, and living room and on condition of 5 hours support time each week I was given my rights and privileges back again. Thanks to Stacy, Ben, Scarlett, Lauren, Alison, Lesley, and Joan (who sadly passed away in 2009, and I continue to remain grateful for all she did for me at Sussex Court) I was able to write my first book and get a whole new life for myself.

Two significant family events occurred in this time. Number One – in June 2007, Chris and Emma got married and I was invited to play keyboard music on the big day. We all flew to Toulouse airport from Leeds/Bradford, and hired a car for the week, which Jonty drove. We went to a wonderful French 'Moulin' where we spent most of our time eating, drinking and relaxing by the swimming pool. Although I fell ill in France, everyone got some good photos and it was a huge family reunion as well with Uncles and Aunts all present. Plus people from America and other countries came especially for the newlyweds.

Secondly, in June 2008, mum had rented a family cottage in the Lake District for a week; 'Scafell View' near Wast Water. We took it in turns to do the cooking, on alternate nights. On my night I made a big beef chow mein with Japanese Sake to drink. There was Mum, Dad, Chris, Emma, Jonny, Jonty, Jenny and myself all present. Jonty and I climbed Great Gable one day, he then ascended Scafell Pike three days in a row, and Chris, Jonty and I did Scafell Pike once. Emma was suffering back problems so she decided it was best to return to base. I couldn't walk for three days afterwards. Several times we went to the local pub for dinner, just a mile down the road. The holiday was a great success and it was very thoughtful for mum to put that on for us all. Thanks mum, love you loads for that!

During this period I had contact with the following friends who were regulars at my flat: Simon Muir, David Ives, Alex Boorman, Katie McNulty, and David Goodwin. Simon came to advise on employment opportunities and talk of his then punk-rock band 'Locust Hotel'. I went out several times to see them in town, before they packed in. Dave 'Ivorias' inspired me to return to piano playing, and I went on to acquire a wonderful Roland piano-keyboard in January 2008, for which I received some 50% financial help from my mum and dad. Dave encouraged my music-making and I even took guitar lessons in Scarborough with Neal Jackson, in Bridlington with Pete Bolton, and in York with John Mackenzie. I attempted to study this instrument from scratch for two years, and acquired some basic skills.

Alex was an 'arranged' friend through the Scarborough Mind circuit. He had been in the army and frequently campaigned for global climate change issues, going to demonstrate in London. He always attended my gigs and spared the time to read my scripts of his own volition. Thanks, mate! Katie was recovering from her own hospital experiences and from a previous relationship with boyfriend Jerome. And David Goodwin – man of the match – was trying to keep me fit and running as he had witnessed the whole marathon bit and we had trained together a lot. David had been very heavy, but continued to train for the Great North Run, and lost over seven stones in weight in the process!

The Green Dragon

With David Ives I was able to have company to attend the annual Scarborough Jazz Festival 2007/08 in the Spa, and the free festival Acoustic Gathering in Peasholm Park 2007/08 as well. There I was astounded by the talent and versatility of the performers. A nurse from hospital was there with her husband so we had a brief chat. Also there was Shona Lloyd from Hull University (during my time there) and several other familiar faces – Ed Beecroft, Alex, Chris Minz et al.

After about a year's practice I was invited to appear in Scarborough Library on piano for a 'MIND fundraiser'. Dave played as principal and I was the guest star that day in 2008. This inspired me to continue into 2009, but with a beautiful addition to my life. In August 2008 I had bumped into Christina in the town centre – the woman I am now married to, whom I had met previously in the year 2000 - she pretty much ran me over with her pram and three young sons. At first we hadn't much to say, but I left my number. A day or so later I received a call from her mum, and then we started communicating more and more. Eventually I went to visit her at home and we determined to stay together from then on. The boys seemed to accept me alright, and as her marriage had fallen through, and I was single, we decided to make up for a very long eight years of lost time.

She supported my music, so in June 2009 I played some classical music at the Saltburn Music Festival coming third, and then again in 2010, coming first in the class with Sinding's 'Rustle of Spring', Chopin's 'Polonaise', Debussy's 'Clair de Lune', and Scott Joplin's 'The Entertainer'. Alex and Dave came to listen in 2009, and Dad, Jonny and Dave in 2010. Christina gave me special permission to go for the evening! Then in August 2009 I played jazz and popular piano in the Marine bar, Whitby. Christina and family came to listen to that too, with Alex sparing half a day for music. My parents also attended. This Whitby gig had been on my mind since March, when Christina and I took a weekend holiday at a quiet cottage near the River Esk via hire car – a Vauxhall Insignia. We made bread, fed the ducks, and walked around Whitby town and discovered the Marine Bar where I wanted to play – and did so some months later. In

September 2009 I joined an acoustic night at Helmsley Arts Centre. Most acts were on guitar, but I did two numbers on piano/vocals. They seemed to go down well enough.

Whilst living in my Sussex Court flat I set up a small lottery syndicate, with five of us playing twice a week. In August 2008 we won four numbers - £120 to split, and over a two year period won £10 about twenty times. We all hoped to win the jackpot, however, so maybe one day?! I attempted to work in London at one point for Rethink, conducting research into interview technique. The prospects were pretty good but I couldn't handle the distance commuting from Scarborough to London and back in the same day. I decided to focus on my music and writing at home.

Since February 2006 I had been involved with the world famous Tony Robbins Seminars in London, and whilst I lived in my flat I attended one UPW (Unleash the Power Within) seminar in June 2007 and one Wealth Mastery seminar in November 2007. These had been a significant focal point for me for a very long time, and the prospects of getting there had meant reason to live whilst being held in hospital. I would like to thank and congratulate Tony Robbins, John Ross, Keith Cunningham, Chuck Mellon, and Joe Williams for their excellence.

More recently, on a more concluding note I would like to wish a fond farewell to 2009, and to Joan Grantham, Michael Jackson, Stephen Gately, Patrick Swazey, and Luciano Pavarotti. May you rest in peace and, God knows, we say thankyou for the music!

Chapter Nine
150 Personal Heroes

The following people are all people to whom I have looked up or revered as heroes in some way at some point in my life. Most are still amongst the living, some I am sorry to say, are no longer, and with an explanation alongside each one, they fall into the following categories:

Family and Friends
Mum and Dad - they have always been there for me through thick and thin, and provided many opportunities during my life for growth and personal development. Thankyou for your love!
Chris Kershaw - my eldest brother; lived and worked in London for over 15 years, always providing free board and lodging whenever I stayed. New York marathon 2000 (3hrs 37mins), and cycled 181km Etape du Tour de France 2010 (10 ½ hours)!
Emma Kershaw, née Maurice – married Chris, and now both live and work in the south of France. Company Director.
Jonty Hakney - cousin; cycled with Chris from Lands End to John O'Groats, French Alps, Spanish Pyrenees, and *regularly* cycles 100s of miles in a typical week.
David Ives   - rekindled my pianistic interests. He has been a great friend too, since 2007. Free hospitality every time!
Simon Muir   - saw me through a difficult few years whilst he formed and sang in Locust Hotel punk-rock band.
Alex Boorman - stuck with me as a friend over the years since 2008 (& Best man).
Sam Belsom   - artist and family friend all my life, cycling, running and swimming.
David Goodwin - fit man, family man and professional actor, regularly appearing on stage and radio.

Music
Jill and David Bowman – Taught me music from an early age, and remain interested in my life to this day. Peace and love to their grown up offspring Jonan and Ruth, living overseas.

Simon Wright - musical maestro of the world. No words are enough for the man!
Michael Jackson - King of Pop (RIP)
Axl Rose - I was a regular fan as a young teen.
Freddie Mercury – same as above.
Billy Joel - The Piano Man!
Elton John - Queen of piano pop.
Rod Stewart - If ya think I'm sexy, come on and tell me so.
Phil Collins - Against all odds, Another day in paradise, In the air tonight, Two worlds, Buster etc. Made the 80's!
Seal - Kiss from a Rose, Crazy, Fast Changes. Mmmm-mmmm
Michael Bolton - That man can sing, like no other. Power ballads are us matey.
Brian May - finger pickin' good dude.
Eric Clapton – Layla, Cream, The Yardbirds, Tears in Heaven.
Yevgeny Kissin - Piano child prodigy, top of the game. Except he's grown up now of course.
Daniel Barenboim - Era of astonishment, excellence, passion, and the lasting loving memory of Jacqueline Du Pre. Pianist, conductor and wonderful man.
Nikolai Demidenko - Russian virtuoso. Mum's hero.
Vladimir Ashkenazy - Jewish virtuoso. I have many recordings in my collection of classics performed by Ashkenazy.
Keith Jarrett – Koln concert 1975. Personal all time favourite piano concert.
Andras Schiff - Bach's 48 Preludes and Fugues. Bartok's concerti. Enough said!
Glenn Gould - Bach, eccentric genius. Went down as rare and unique virtuoso. I tried to locate Gould's studio when I visited Toronto, Canada.
Angela Hewitt - Bach's 48 Preludes and Fugues.
Nicki Isles - Jazz giant of our era. Met once on a London jazz workshop weekend.
Toots Thielmans - Harmonica wizard.
George Shearing - love the jazz arrangements for piano.
Thelonius Monk - unstoppable dexterity and virtuosity.
Duke Ellington - player with love.
Nat King Cole – Crooner and pianist.

Pascal Rogé - collected recordings and attended one live concert at Settrington Orangery.

Sports
Lance Armstrong - Seven times Tour de France winner.
Bernard Hinault, Eddie Mercx, Jacques Anquetil – all five times Tour de France winners.
Ian Botham - Met once at charity fishing weigh-in. He congratulated the winner.
Damon Hill - Formula One Champion.
Nigel Mansall - Formula One Champion.
Jensen Button - Formula One Champion.
Louis Hamilton - *The* Formula One Champion.
Jonny Wilkinson - Won World Cup Rugby for GB 2003.
Michael Phelps - 8 Olympic Golds at Beijing for swimming.
Paula Radcliffe - London and New York marathon winner.
Kenenisa Bekele - Distance Running Champion – World and Olympic titles.
Linford Christie - Olympic champion sprinter, once the world's fastest man.
Usain Bolt - Current World Record Holder 100m, 200m and 4 * 100m relay Jamaican Team Olympic Golds at Beijing 2008.
Kelly Holmes - Double Olympic Champion Athens 2004 (800m, 1500m).
Sally Gunnell - Olympic Champion 400m hurdles
Jonathan Edwards - World record holder and Olympic Champion triple jumper.
Steve Cram - Olympic medallist 800m and 1500m. World Champion runner of the 80's. He came to talk to Durham school running club in 1996.
Steve Ovett - Champion distance runner in the same league.
Sebastian Coe - 1980 Olympic champion Gold medallist 800m, 1500m. Lord Coe is now in charge of the London 2012 Olympic Games.
Stephen Hendry - Snooker multi- world champion
Ronnie O'Sullivan – created fastest ever 147 break in under 5 minutes. I read his autobiography as he keeps winning all the titles.

Ken Doherty   - 1997 World Snooker Champion.
John Higgins   - 21st Century Snooker World Champion.
Marco Fu   - World Class snooker player
Paul Hunter   - RIP Yorkshire's finest snooker player.
Jimmy White   - Ambassador of snooker, and Jungle Celebrity VIP. Always a gentleman!
Steven Lee   - Snooker class A.
Sean Murphy   - Snooker champion from the North East.

Authors
Steven R Covey - The 7 habits became the eighth habit.
Bill Bryson   - travel comedy genius. I have read all his books.
Nick Hornby   - again, a complete genius. Really glad they turned his work into film.
J R R Tolkien - Lord of The Rings, The Silmarillion, Children of Hurin, The Hobbit et al. Wonderful.
Stephen Fry   - much ado about the tv; there is too much to say here.

Students (Durham School)
Marc Burton   - 1st xv rugby captain.
Alistair Lowe   - Head of house.
Gareth Blackbird – Head of school.
Andrew Lowes   - Determined to join the army.
Megan Ellis   - beautiful and multi-talented.
Barney Ellis   - big brother of above and talented.
Rupert Ellis   - brother of above; we share the same birthday.
Matthew Courtney – RIP my most incredible friend. I remember Matthew for being the best at everything he ever did.
Christopher Hilton – Head of school.
Diccon Humphrey   - dated Liberty Kidd.
William Bishop   - won the Dunelmian 10 mile run.
Edwin James   - a Nationals standard runner, won every race he entered at Durham school.
Aidan Adams   - County runner and Nationals skier.
Andrew Turner - inspiring rugby seven's captain.

Teachers
Hugh Dias   - in loco parentis for my 5 Durham years.
Mark Bushnell - Economics Master and athletics coach. Both the above offered sponsorship when I ran my marathon in 2006.
Derek Best   - Assistant Headmaster. Supported my speech and voted in my favour contrary to many of my student peers.
Michael Lang   - Headmaster; gave me 5 good Durham Years
Mr Dougal   - Athletics coach, and married Kim Hamilton (ex-Triathlete and taught me GCSE PE).
Tim Chapman - French teacher, rugby and cross country coach.
John Hamer   - Latin, Maths, cricket, referee, comedian!
Martin Wright - History, PE, and Sports coaching.
Ken Starks   - Sciences, and taught me Chopsticks on piano.
Jo Malia   - Art, and led expedition to Crianlarich, Scotland. One training incident on night walk where our campsite was blown severely by high winds.
Fred Cook   - CDT, cross country, and loved his family.
David Crook   - 'The Boss', rugby, French, Spanish, and organised trips abroad.
Nick Vise   - rugby, French, Spanish and a loving father.
Roger Muttit   - Director of Music.
Diane Evans   - Biology teacher and ambassador
Mr Burgess   - Head of Biology, also Crianlarich leader.

Mentors/Life Coaches
Jesus   - his life was sacrificed to save the people; I wear a neck-crucifix to remind me of his love every day.
Tony Robbins   - he's written about it, dedicated his life to teaching about it and regularly appears in front of thousands of followers to learn about it. Being the best you can be.
Andrew Matthews   - author, cartoonist, seminarist, leader. Both the above two became extraordinarily wealthy as a consequence of their success, happiness, and life improvement movements. I read their books and attended 3 Robbins seminars 2006-07. I got from them what I had perceived as right for me.
Dr Joe Vitale – Enlightened Healer and life coach. NB 'The Secret' & 'The Missing Secret'

Tony Smith – Malton housemate with a genial mind and character
Matthew Havenhand - My social worker, who understands all.
Dr Mogyorosy   - My Doctor, who understands all.
Dr Nicholson   - Ditto the above

Politicians
Al Gore - Runner-up to George W Bush 2004.
John Kerry   - Runner-up to George W Bush 2000. On both occasions I had hoped that these two men would be elected.

Presidents
Barack Obama   - US President elect 2008 +. Michelle, Sasha and Malia, All-American First Family.
Bill Clinton   - US President 1990's. Hilary and Chelsea always a boost for him. Wrote 'Giving', 2008.
Nicholas Sarkozy   - Presents as younger, experienced and a French Treasure.
Jacques Chirac   - Diamant Brillant!
Koffi Annan   - UN Secretary-General, fixing matters of import around the world.
John F Kennedy - Saw Neil Armstrong land on the moon in his era. Helped cause the Berlin Wall to come down after his speech, 'Ich bin ein Berliner'.

Prime Ministers
David Cameron - Conservative coalition PM with Nick Clegg (Lib Dems).
Gordon Brown   - UK 2008 + made equal opportunities for all.
Tony Blair   - UK 1997 New Labour party formed. Stuck with Cheri throughout Premiership.
Paul Martin   - Canadian ex PM 2004. I visited the residence in Ottawa on my travels.
Margaret Thatcher   - The Iron Lady, regulated a sturdy Britain

Movie Stars
Timothy Spall   - Auf Wiedersehen Pet, The Last Samurai.
Gary Sinise   - Forrest Gump, CSI New York.

The Green Dragon

Tom Hanks — Forrest Gump, Saving Private Ryan, Big, etc…
Jean Claude van Damme - Bloodsports
Jackie Chan - he's funny, he fights, and he can act
Bruce Lee - Enter the Dragon.
Steven Seagal - Navy Seals
Arnold Schwarzenegger - Governor of California, -post movies
Danny Devito - Twins
Leonardo di Caprio - Romeo and Juliet, Titanic, Blood Diamond, The Beach. Icon of the age.

Sean Connery
Roger Moore
George Lazenby
Timothy Dalton } The authentic James Bond 007's
Daniel Craig 'Shaken not stirred'!
Pearce Brosnan

TV Personalities

Anne Robinson - The Weakest Link, Watchdog. Never misses a beat, quick to catch a blinking eye, and very rude.
Michael Parkinson - Chat show host whose shows I enjoyed for years.
Jonathan Ross - Chat show comedian, film guru.
Richard Whiteley - RIP Countdown's original host.
Dermot O'Leary
Simon Cowell
Louis Walsh
Danii Minogue } The X Factor judges/hosts, thankyou!
Cheryl Cole
Sharon Osbourne
Jack Osbourne - Ozzy, Sharon, Jack, Kelly, famous family

Chefs

Gordon Ramsay - Hell's Kitchen, The F word, no nonsense.

Jamie Oliver   - '15' restaurants, The Naked Chef, Global outreach, and Sainsbury's; love him!
Ainsley Harriott - Ready Steady Cook!
Nigella Lawson - Extraordinary chef with delightful recipes.
Delia Smith   - One of the all time greats in UK cooking.
Anthony Warrell Thompson – fun, and exquisite culinary skills.
James Martin – trained in Scarborough, my hometown.

Comedians
Michael Macintyre   - very funny indeed
Lee Evans   - Hilariously clued up comedy
Jack Dee   - also Big Brother winner. Makes me laugh.
Dara O'Briain   - Mock the Week and absolutely clued-up comedy.
Morecambe and Wise   - Dad's Christmas favourites for decades.
Boris Johnson   - Lord Mayor of London. Best look out!

*

The list could go on to include Dr Who's, and many other noteworthy people but mainly I would like to express profound gratitude to those listed for all the joy and meaning they have brought me in my life. A very warm thankyou indeed!

Chapter Ten
Family

This closing chapter, entitled 'Family', ranges from my originally being the youngest member of the family, with two older brothers and my parents around, to today, when I am the oldest member of another household, with Christina, the twins and three older boys. This transition will be elaborated on here.

On 29th September, 2009, I was in Scarborough Hospital with Christina. Her pregnancy had reached the 37th week (of 40) and the midwives had decided to induce the twins around 11 o'clock that morning. Their decision had been made some weeks previously, however, so we came prepared. Having spent the earlier part of the morning driving by the seaside and around the castle headland driveway, Christina said that she was ready for the birth process, and I admired her courage and bravery already.

We got to the hospital about 9am and made our way into the antenatal ward with our bags. She was very calm throughout but I was beginning to sweat and feel nervous for her, although I knew that she had been there before for her three older boys. I wanted to be there when it mattered most. We were due twin boys. I had been with Christina for every outpatient appointment during the pregnancy, and made sure to get her what was needed. We had use of a hire car as well, which helped. In fact by the time that 2009 had ended we had hired a car over five times throughout the year! Today we own our very own Vauxhall Zafira, courtesy of winning some money in the People's Postcode Lottery in September 2010. We started planning our wedding, and sort out the things we have meant to for a long time – including getting a car, and paying off our immediate debts etc. This came a year after the twins were born though, so they saw their first birthday shortly after our windfall.

The midwife invited us to enter a smaller room where the induction would occur. A surgeon appeared with the equipment to give Christina an epidural injection into her spine to numb the pain. Also, there was a 'gas and air' combination (oxygen and Entonox) which helped her feel a bit more comfortable. This breathing apparatus produced a kind of 'high' sensation – I know because I was given some in a relaxed moment. The process was beginning to turn surreal, ie 'can this actually be happening?'

Guess what – it really was happening and faster by the minute! Shortly after this Christina was wheeled into the operating theatre and I was invited to be there for the birth, although the doctors never made me wear a gown or medical cloak. I wore my orange jumper that Christina had seen me put on that morning back at home. It helped. I couldn't help but admire Christina's courage. She was magnificent throughout the entire procedure! In the theatre room were approximately ten midwives, doctors and nurses, plus myself and Christina. Each had a specific role to play.

That afternoon at 12.35pm and 12.45pm, the twins were born, entering the world with a huge cry. Both babies were relieved of their umbilical cords and then placed in a special birth-cot. So, two beautiful, natural-born twins arrived.

I simply wish to say 'thankyou' to Christina for bearing our twin boys. They are the world to me. At the time of birth Christina was not sure whether to give them her surname, or mine - 'Kershaw', but the hospital ruled that we give the mother's name on the birth bands around their ankles, until their registered birth certificates; so for a day they were 'Stephensons', until they were registered on their birth certificates as 'Kershaws'.

There were many visitors whilst Christina was in hospital. Mum bought her flowers, her sister bought her clothes for the twins, and her Aunty bought clothes, too, for the twins. I had visited H Samuels for a token gift to give to Christina to say thankyou. I bought her a truth charm bracelet with five lucky charms attached – a love heart, a mini pram, lucky horsehoe, lucky star, and a locket for a photo. She received many gifts from various family members after the birth, and more flowers from me and the next-door-neighbours, too, who had been looking after me in the evenings back home, making me free meals for a week (Brett and Joan). At that time we lived in the Barrowcliffe area, on St Leonard's Crescent, where I had moved in with Christina. Once the twins became 6 months old we qualified for a bigger house in the Newby area of Scarborough, where we live today, a 3 bedroom semi-detached house with living room, dining room, shed-utility room, kitchen, bathroom and garden. We were offered a Springer Spaniel called Roxy from Christina's brother-in-law, and sister. She accepted Roxy gladly, so there was a crowded house and much ado from then on for us both.

Suddenly there I was – husband, father and step-dad. My life had just changed enormously. My biggest ever challenge had just arrived – would I be able to live up to all this? The next day I placed an announcement in the local Evening News to welcome the twins, and to express my gratitude, with love to Christina, of course. A brand new turn, two new born lives to love and bring up. Could I do this? Could I be a great dad?

For the next six days there would be continuous hospital visits every day. There were countless visitors to see the babies as well. Christina had a look in her eyes as if to say 'There, I told you I could do this!' She seemed happier, especially as she learnt that another recent birth had been stillborn. After all she has ever been through, Christina deserved the happiness of her loving children. The eldest two know this instinctively. The older boys are eight, six, and three and very protective of their mother – and she of them.

Suddenly I had my first significant role to play in a family. I was no longer the baby boy, the son and brother. I was Dad! Here are a couple of poems I wrote for our twins about the time of their birth:

Soon to be
Held in our hearts dear
Two little boys
Who require lots of toys

Jamie Kershaw

Cameron and Oliver
There may be a sleepless night
Crying from a fright
Discrepancy in spite

Of the love we share
The clothes we all wear
And shelter above our hair
I like my layer

Cameron and Oliver
Olly and Cam
Come along now
Let the world know you're no sham

I love you Christina
The boys know this
Together we grow keener
And I mean it when we kiss!

Also, I wrote the following poem:

Two blessed boys
Filled with good grace
Fortune in their favour

Two blessed boys
Coming from God above
I love you one and all

With Christina by my side
And the Eternal as my guide
Our family does strive

To go on and through
The daily to-do
Olly hello – Cam too

What is this world, this life

The Green Dragon

If we cannot produce
My love is for you. XxX

I did ask for a miracle in my life some years ago, and now here they are – two beautiful boys. Sometimes miracles do happen after all!

All I knew was that my own Mum and Dad had been there for me my whole life, through thick and thin. Whenever I did need them they would be there for me. Their opportunities ranged over the years from one thing to another, but some of the more exciting events that I can recall included a London boat trip on the river Thames, and a tour to see the Beefeaters in the Tower of London, guarding Her Majesty's crown jewels. Also, a view of Buckingham Palace through the railings, and Trafalgar Square with the bronze lions and the thousand pigeons. I was just three when we three boys were taken up to Scotland by train for a week's camping by Loch Torridon. Closer to home they took us boys to the theme parks at Flamingo Land and Lightwater Valley on several occasions; holidays to Nottingham – Sherwood Forest Centre Parc; musicals, plays and cinema trips including West Side Story, Macbeth (at Sheriff Hutton Castle), Christmas pantomime, and Fantasia. In York City she took us to magic shows/shops and often to the Early Learning Centre to buy toys. Also, every June, for the longest day of the year, we would all go camping on the moors by 'Losky Beck', and stay up late to see the daylight at 11 pm. Mum would take us for a midnight walk.

By the age of ten, Jonny and I owned our very own computer - a Commodore 64 with games including Pitstop, Paradroid, Run the Gauntlet, Last Ninja 2, The Summer Games, etc. Amazing to think that these days the XBox, and Wii evolved via Nintendo Gameboy. Many of the boys here have a Nintendo DS to play on. Christina's brother-in-law and sister gave a DS and Wii to their kids, one boy got a DS this last Christmas, and I believe that Christina's other sister and brother-in-law gave their boys a Nintendo DS to play as well. Now they all have X-Boxes and Wii's!

My own parents also took us on trips further afield over the years, ranging from Cornwall to see Uncle Rob, Aunty Wendy, Matthew, and Helen. Also, Uncle Andy, Aunty Ricky, Christiana, and Antonia in Worcestershire, en route. These tended to be summer vacations for the family every year. I especially remember the Trethowa days – they were the best, involving swimming pool, Ben the dog, tractor lawnmower, and Redwing boat for mackerel fishing. These days, Matthew is married to Holly and they have two sons – Arlo and Otto. Matthew worked over the years as chef, ski instructor, surf instructor, beach manager, and Head chef too. Helen's eldest son is called Jordan. Antonia went to the Nationals as a cyclist and even got to compete in the World Championships in Pakistan recently. Christiana studied medicine at Cambridge and works full time towards being a consultant anaesthetist. Uncle Rob moved again after about ten years, to Devon. A village called 'Holcombe Rogus', where I once cut their lawn on a tractor lawnmower. Then, after so many years, he decided to return to Cornwall – 'Bolitho's Cottage' near Helston where he and Wendy have remained to this day, along with Helen, Matthew and grandchildren also in Cornwall to visit them, maybe sometimes.

We also visited France (Paris, River Seine, barge trip 1991 with the Bowmans) and skiing at Val D'Isere from Terrington with Mum and others. We met the pilot on the flight home and were presented with badges. Another skiing holiday with mum was to Austria – the Pitztal Glacier – with Jonny, too, and met colleagues Tom Williams and Jenny Elm (whose wedding I attended in 2008 – not to Tom though!). When my mum's parents lived in Spain, we flew there for Christmas or summer holidays, but I was too young to really remember any of that now. There were some friends living in Scotland, near Fort William, but I can't remember the details now, just the fact that we visited on occasion. Other trips to Bonny Scotland were to the Edinburgh military tattoo with Daniel Utley and his father, Mr Julian Utley (then an ITV cameraman). That was when I was still at Terrington.

The Green Dragon

Later on, a post-Durham New Year party was spent at the Edinburgh Hogmanay. In a nutshell, I was due to meet friends but our meeting didn't happen, so I was just a face in the crowd that night, 1998-99. I hitchhiked back to York on New Year's Day having spent all my money on the night out. Several familiar faces did pop up though, whilst I was there, such as Elliott Brown, Simon Reay and their girlfriends. They were going to see the band called 'Texas' doing a gig. I'm sure I saw Emily Geiser in the crowd that night, too, also from Durham School. Other New Year's eves, for most of my life, have been spent watching Jools Holland's Hootenanny on TV. I enjoyed the showmanship of the artists concerned. The majority of Christmases have been spent with Mum, Dad, Jonny and Chris at home, eating turkey and opening our gifts from under the tree. Once, when Chris first moved to London, Jonny and I joined him for a London Christmas. Another year, later on, I was in Canada for Christmas, and then a few years after that I shared two family Christmas with Christina's family in Scarborough, as well as going to see Mum and Dad.

When I was 14 I went on summer holiday with a Durham School friend - Andy Millson. We went to Ibiza on a family holiday. The details are in an earlier chapter, though. We came back tanned and more worldly-wise!

Mum also took us boys to Harrogate Dry Ski Slope and Ripon Sailing Club at different times. She owned an Enterprise called Crumpet and a Mirror Dingy. I once was given a small boat which I called Red Gremlin. This didn't last too long and I never got into sailing much anyway. We were capsized by a freak storm one time and that put me off, I reckon.

Mum's cooking is definitely one of her assets in life. She could invent recipes and write an entire recipe book if she wanted. I would buy a copy, and I am sure that Delia Smith would take notes from her! I used to watch her cook and learnt some basics that way. Please refer to the forthcoming list for my staple diet of the last ten years.

However, Mum's greatest satisfaction has to be from running Helmsley Arts Centre. Originally it had been a Quaker Meeting House, called the Old Meeting House, and she and a few friends bought the disused building and turned it into a performing arts centre. Over twenty years later, with multiple patrons, constant expansion and development, and one great fire, the place is a successful, thriving, buzzing, international venue, and the waiting list is so long that many perfectly likely performances have to be turned down in the selection process. Mum actually hired out the HAC bar for her family one Christmas. Chris and Emma came from France and I was there with Christina and three of the boys. We had a good time.

That list, by the way, of survival food for the cookbook; Gordon Ramsay would probably tell me to go wear an f-ing creative hat, and goodness knows what Jamie Oliver would say, but I have appreciated recipes for the following meals since the age of 19, when self-catering began for me:

Spaghetti bolognese, shepherd's pie, chilli con carne, mince-onion and mash potato, avocado chicken grill, curries including Rogan Josh-Dansak-Biryani-Korma-Madras (Lamb, King prawn, Chicken, Vegetable), tomato-lentil soup, leek and potato soup, vegetable soup, chicken chow mein, paella, kidney bean-onion-tomato-cheese bake, spinach-chick-pea-tuna and lemon, pasta twirls with bacon-pepper-or tuna, bruschetta, pizzas, full English breakfast (when my Dad makes them they are then 'World Famous Fry-ups), stuffed mushrooms, stuffed peppers, ham salad, ploughman's lunch, chicken soup, chicken risotto, kedgeree, smoked mackerel salad, quiches, Sunday roasts, steak-chips-peas, sausage casserole, burger-chips-beans, sausage-red onion gravy-mashed potato, sandwiches, pickled eggs, home-baked bread, cheesecake, chococrispies, flapjacks, biscuits, cakes (homemade coffee-chocolate-lemon-strawberry-fruit), yogurts, ice cream and jelly. This has been my main diet for a very long time.

We have always been food fans. Moving onto the next family story, I would like to mention Chris and Emma – my eldest

The Green Dragon

brother and sister-in-law. Chris left York Sixth form college aged 18 with A-levels in Economics, Sociology and Information Technology and decided to move straight to London to find work after a cycling tour of New Zealand with college friend Mike Edison who is now a practising lawyer on the verge of moving to New Zealand with wife and baby daughter. He had also cycled from York to Istanbul with college friend Ed, learning Esperanto on the way and visiting Esperantists in the Czech Republic, Bulgaria, and Turkey. Another college friend whom Chris keeps in touch with is Dave.

Over a fifteen year period, Chris had over ten addresses in London, and began work as a park gardener when he first moved. Then came work at Oddbins off-licences as a shop-assistant and delivery driver. This lasted for many years, and at some point Chris determined to go to Middlesex University to read English and Information Technology. He kept fit and in 2000 ran the New York marathon in 3hrs 37mins. Whilst at Middlesex he established a running club, and came out with a 2.1 for his degree! As a result of his new qualification, he applied for better-paid office work and for a period of approximately one year worked in a city office, but in the end wanted to be self-employed, somehow. How to do this? Chris knew what he wanted, so undertook trade courses in carpentry. His 'apprenticeship' lasted quite a while. I even helped once on a job by chance invitation whilst in London. He had found his niche now, and after another few changes of address, he met Emma, initially as a work acquaintance in the wine business, and over many years they got to know each other, until one day they somehow "clicked". Chris and Emma never looked back, as they had both independently lived and worked in London for a very long time. Emma had also lived and worked in Paris for some years, prior to meeting Chris.

They decided to move together into a lovely house in West Norwood, where they stayed for at least another three years. Chris, by now, had his own carpentry workshop and business enterprise up and running, and Emma directed some major wine business all around the country. Somehow they still managed to have time for people like me, and often cycled out to Brighton for the day. Emma's sister Liza married Steve and they have two boys Ben and Thomas. Her other sister, Claire, lives in America with husband Brock, son Oliver, and daughter Mia. As far as I am aware her parents live in Chalfont St Peter, Bucks. Her father had been in the Navy in earlier years, and I had the privilege of meeting them when, in June 2007, I was invited to be at Chris and Emma's wedding in the South of France. They had asked me to play piano-keyboard on their big day, with Dad on clarinet. My biggest appearance ever!

Today, Chris and Emma live and work in the South of France. They moved in 2008. I was invited out one time so went to their converted barn for a week. It's funny how you can feel close to family even though so far away, or after so many events come between times. Life's river flows on! They moved into a house in a village called La Serpent, then to Coustouge, where they are building their own home today (2011). A very bold, enterprising move! When I visited, Chris had work in a small town called Montreal. He asked me to help out with a fitting and varnishing job over two days, so I did. We visited the local market and I was left to my own devices for a while, so I kept texting Christina to make me feel better.

Christina and I have been together for two years now since 2008, but we knew each other since 2000 as mentioned previously. My trip to France was a bit risky though, because it meant leaving Christina for a week at an early stage in our relationship. Just before I left we decided to buy a cute little puppy dog (a golden yellow Labrador) whom we named Charlie. One morning we got in a taxi with two of the boys to go to Burniston kennels to look at the puppy dogs. Within an hour we were on the way home with Charlie and two excited boys. I was excited, too – I had wanted my own pet dog since I was seven. So, 23 years of waiting for what turned out to be a four-month event.

While I was gone for the week, Christina had her three boys and Charlie at home. We had agreed that I would phone on an evening and write as well. My constant communications upset

The Green Dragon

Chris and Emma a little, so my trip was not that great. I was glad to get home to Christina, the boys, and Charlie the dog. We learnt that babies and puppies are not compatible, though. Lots of jumping, pooing on carpets, tearing, chewing and other curious behaviour – sometimes scaring the boys as well. To keep it brief, we had a disagreement and couldn't keep Charlie any longer, so after about four months I called a taxi and took Charlie back to the kennels where he had come from. I cried. For the first time in many years. It hurt to have to do that. Really a lot!

Post-Charlie days, it is now a year on, and we are still together doing fine with our family. We have our moments but I have come to learn that, despite the discontent and differences of opinion I do love Christina, and that is why I asked her to marry me. I even asked her parents beforehand. We are as one. Most days go by and we are hardly apart for more than four hours at any time. That would be on a trip to town or to see the family, or even to have time apart when we need to calm down a little. Since the twins were born we have been on an alternating schedule where one sleeps in bed and the other stays up with the babies all night. The downside is we hadn't shared our bed for over three months, except for a fleeting cuddle, or a lie down. I looked forward to the day when we could spend a night together again. This occurred more frequently after the babies became six – nine months old. They are now two years old!

I have learnt rather quickly that looking after a four year old is not something that comes without difficulties. I have learnt that I am not the centre of the universe after all. The six year old is! And doesn't he like to make it known! Everything revolves around him in our home. That's the beauty of it. He is the big brother whilst the other two stay with their Dad and Nana, so whilst he is the oldest boy he is happy. The twins quadrupled in weight in their first two years, going from about 5lb, to 20lb in weight. A healthy development. By now they both smiled and grinned independently at Christina and me. Either that or covered us in poo and puke. Oliver can say 'Mama', and 'Dada', has beautiful blue eyes and crawls fast. Cameron has said 'Mama', has brown eyes and now has two teeth.

For the last five years social services have been coming and going in my life, and it was said that we could be entitled to apply for a three or four bedroom house, owing to overcrowding. So, to move house would make our living space a whole lot more comfortable. We moved into a three bedroom house, with modern kitchen, dining room, utility room/shed outhouse, living room, bathroom, and garden. That was a dream come true, until we had to separate and see each other at contact times during the week.

In a nutshell, I would like to be here for Christina where it most matters. I know that she deserves love and support from me. She gets plenty from the family already. If I can at least show willing and lend a hand, then at least I'm showing an interest. I know we love each other. And that's a lot, that's enough for me. I also know that in previous experiences Christina has had a hard time, and people have caused her upset and grief. I would like to replace those negative experiences with my love and try to establish a happier, more positive relationship between the two of us and our boys.

I am now a kind of 'step-Dad' and I find it interesting that I can relate to the boys on equal footing. I know my own inner child, and we often have fun and games and outings as a family, though I find it very hard to discipline them, or get them to calm down when carried away. This happens a lot. Sadly in February this year, I couldn't cope with the pressures anymore and one morning I was being very lazy and laying late in bed on a Sunday, and something snapped inside of me. After many months of usually walking away when upset, I actually hit Christina that morning; more an actual beating. I was arrested and taken into Police custody for the day. Christina was seriously hurt and had to go to Hospital for a check up as she was badly bruised. It took about two weeks for the bruises to disappear again; meanwhile social services came along and after much deliberation we had to live apart, with me living in

The Green Dragon

Beadlam with Mum and Dad, and Christina living in Newby with the boys. Fortunately, having the car meant visits were possible, and with the agreement of social services, we are currently on five days a week, and healing faster every day together, seeing the boys whenever possible. I know that I want as much to do with my wife and kids as possible, and they with me. Time will tell...

Christina's other two sons are from her previous marriage. I have been glad to help out at the house when they are around and I think that they have accepted me by now. Occasionally they call me 'dad' in their utterances, but usually follow this with 'Jamie', 'Lollipop', 'Bitscitz' (Biscuit), or 'Bot-bots' (bottle). The eldest is probably happy to get the extra Christmas presents, and both boys came to visit my parents a couple of times, which involved a long bus ride to get there and back again. I feel to have taken on the boys as part of my own life now and hope that I can provide for everyone. The boys have taken to piano and guitar with me on occasion, opting to play 'their own style'.

Christina often 'wears the trousers' at home and corrects me when I say something unacceptable, or sit around too long. We do have a laugh together every so often, and one evening in December, the boys were all being looked after, so the two of us went out for a curry in The Indian Rose Brasserie. That was the only time the two of us have been out together during our relationship, and I enjoyed it very much.

Another favourite venue for going out is the kids' Playzone. The two eldest love it there, and often ask to go back. It doesn't cost too much and gives the kids the physical space to cavort and run around as much as they want.

It is thanks to one family member that I was offered a spot to play piano, for experience, in the Grand Hotel in Scarborough. He was Hotel Porter, and at the time put in a word to the Manager! Also, they came to listen when I played piano in Whitby Marine Bar in August 2009. I am grateful for their time.

I have to confess that for the last four years I have been an occasional smoker, sometimes buying a box of ten which would typically last over a week. I started with Menthol but now tend to go for Mayfair or Richmond. This habit was once spat upon by myself as I couldn't stand smoking – the smell even made me ill, but since the Social Services forced their way into my life I picked up cigarettes.

Also, drinking Red Bull has occurred on a daily basis since I got together with Christina. She loves this drink and freely encourages its consumption, as it has high caffeine content. We often eat one main meal a day on an evening. Since we got together my life has changed from free man doing whatever I choose, to regulated father being closely monitored every move. Sometimes it's hard to adjust. We alternated sleep nights whilst the babies were still very young, so at least we got sleep on a regular basis. Things calmed down once again since the twins were born. I am often happy enough with my music and writing, although this doesn't always appeal to Christina.

In the meantime we both used Facebook to talk with friends around the world. So far I have over 200 friends from as far away as Australia, Mexico, Germany, Spain, Sweden, Denmark, New York, and the Netherlands. Maybe I owe somebody something somewhere along the line.

Musically I have played a lot of piano privately over the years, but since 2008 I have given the following gigs:- Scarborough library (piano guest at a charity concert for Mind), Saltburn Music Festival pianist (3rd place 2009/1st place 2010), Helmsley Arts Centre Acoustic Night (2 songs), Whitby Marine Piano Bar (guest pianist), Scarborough Westborough Church (Janine's Life Exhibition in Art and Music), and the Scarborough Grand Hotel (mentioned earlier). If it wasn't for meeting David Ives I probably would not have picked the piano up again after all that time out.

Writing-wise, I completed 'Plan 103f' in April 2009 and Chipmunkapublishing generously offered to publish the work.

The Green Dragon

Later in the year, one boy saw this folder on a shelf and asked me about the 'friendly green dragon'. I asked which one – did he mean the model dragon on the desk? He told me he meant the folder with the book in it. 'The Green Dragon' was thus chosen to be the title for this book – my autobiography, hopefully ready this year (2011). It is the story of my life so far.

Birthdays have always been a big thing. When I was growing up I liked to be remembered every year. Also, for the boys here, there are often parties or gatherings put on for them all for a birthday. House visits are regular events between family members every week in one way or another.

Talking of house visits, I haven't been through to Bradford for a long time to see cousin Jonty. We used to meet up regularly, as he did gardening for Mum and Dad in Beadlam. During the year I would go through to his place several times for a night and some nourishment. Whilst at Hull I once went to Bradford to train with Jonty – hill training. I ran on foot, he showed me the route on his bike. I remember we covered about 10 miles one morning, en route to running my one-time-only marathon. The session was a good one and the weather cold and damp, but it wasn't raining.

Jonty inherited his mum's house – my late Aunty Jean. She got cancer in her 60's and Dad was left really hurt (her brother) when she passed on. Dad used to call her 'Kid' even though she was four years older. Whenever we had a family visit to Bradford, Aunty Jean would always put on a huge spread for all of us. Jonty used to show us boys his military collection of rifles, camouflage, and model soldiers – all hand-painted.

His father – my Uncle Frank – died peacefully of old age in April 2011, at home. He had divorced Aunty Jean, though I never know the details, and moved to Beverley with his second wife, Maureen. Jenny – Jonty's sister – also lives in West Yorkshire, and sometimes meets up with Dad and us lot for a social gathering, such as the Lake District cottage, June 2008. It had been many years since I'd seen Jenny, so it was good to be there all together for a change. I attended his funeral with mum and dad. Jonty made a tribute, and Jenny was really upset. There were quite a number of his former friends and Cambridge colleagues present, as he had been a Cambridge Philosopher in his youth.

Nana and Grandpa both passed on during the 1990's after living at 308 Kings Road, Bradford all of my Dad's life. He often took us to visit them in their later years. They never moved until the time came for them to move into old-folks' homes. Dad saw everything! Grandpa played banjo and guitar very well, and Nana was a hobby artist. Mum's parents lived at 8 Leadbetter Drive, in Bromsgrove, near Birmingham, for a long time after they came home from Spain. I used to enjoy our visits there – especially as there was a huge park nearby to play, exercise, Frisbee, ball and mess around in. I did their garden once but got carried away so wasn't allowed to garden next time we visited. Mum was extremely upset when her parents passed on in their later years. I was still at school so didn't know what she was going through at the time.

My mum has been through a lot! A very lot! Her sister, Margaret, died in her twenties, then Jonny and I born by caesarean, then our troubled teens and periods of illness, and the loss of her parents. On top of all that she managed to raise a family and make her dreams come true. Helmsley Arts Centre owes its success to her. Her family owe it to her. There are lots of people whose lives she has reached out to over the years.

Dad celebrated his 80th birthday on 30th May 2011! The day was literally a smashing occasion, as he opened a bottle of champagne and, despite warnings to move the bottle, the cork blasted out and smashed the kitchen strip light into a thousand pieces! After a moment's incredulity, we looked at each other, then to the glass, then to the bottle of fizz, and suddenly all burst out laughing hysterically for quite some time! A day to remember.

The Green Dragon

Jonny would be lost if it wasn't for mum. He was the most intelligent one of us, the fastest runner, and the best musician, along with being a dare-devil on a motorbike. Then suddenly things got on top of him. His friend Jo Crook died in a caravan fire, and another, Ben Rochford, died young from a condition, and Jonny then lost interest in many things. To this day he plays guitar better than many, and enjoys nothing more than a night out eating and drinking in York. If it wasn't for Jonny, I would also have struggled over the years. I often stayed overnight at his place in York, or joined his friends for a night out, though I struggled to get into the scene. I love my brother Jonny, his art is good, he can be funny, and always picks up the phone when I call!

One of Jonny's lifelong friends, Sam Belsom, also crossed paths with my life at various points. When I was running a lot, I think he felt inspired to do the same, because he went on to complete the Kirbymoorside, Helmsley and Castle Howard 10kms some time later, when I went to watch and cheer him on. Sam has been a potter, an artist, a driver, a gardener, charity volunteer, Uncle and brother (Toby is his elder brother, Oliver his nephew), and he is an extremely affable man. He never puts anyone down or says a bad word about anyone. I used to admire his artwork and guitar attempts. Once, Mum drove us all the way to Staffordshire so I could look round Keele University and Sam could buy a pottery wheel. That was a long day trip!

Another family friend over the years has been David Goodwin. David is an actor by trade, calling himself 'Dominic' professionally, husband to Rose, and father to Danny and Katie. In 1998 I had a bit-part as the 'Wall' in Midsummer Night's Dream alongside him. That was the first and last acting appearance I ever made on Helmsley stage! Eight years later, David continues acting on Tours and always has the main part to play, eg Frankenstein, and routinely appears on local radio too. Following a fitness regime in 2007-08, we used to go running together on local routes. This training partnership lasted about two years, and we covered 10km regularly. David went on to do the Great North Run several times, and still looks forwards to the next time round. We ran cross-country at Ampleforth, and did some road running, moorland running, and coastal running around Scarborough Headland. My running became roller-blading, then cycling, then walking, and except when we get in the car – then we drive!

Also Joe Beckett from near Beadlam, just got married to a beautiful Cambodian lady this summer (2011) and they have a young son whom I met with the twins earlier this summer. Years ago Joe and I went for a pint together – Joe went on to work as an assistant for Trekforce in Central America, and found work in his new homeland of Cambodia in finance. We were both pleased to meet again after all those years and change of circumstances!

So, there we have it – thanks to a thousand and one people (maybe more) – my life story so far. I would like to conclude with the words that one can always improve, but what has mattered most of all to me has been the lessons I have learnt, the grace of a kind word or thought shared from another person, whether spoken or written. And of course, I would like to reiterate my gratitude to my Mum and Dad for all the love and opportunities they have provided me with over the years. May your grandchildren do you proud, may you feel fulfilled with life well spent, may your love be known. Thankyou!

The Green Dragon

Postscript

Three pieces for the postscript are firstly, Music of the Millennium, secondly my current CV, and thirdly, the letter to Rethink when I moved out of the Sussex Court flat and handed in my keys.

Music of the Millennium (1990-2010)

This chapter will look into my experiences and explorations of music, since the age at which music first started to make sense to me, to the present day. Whether music by participation or music by appreciation – it all counted!

My experiences with contemporary music began round about 1990, aged 10-12, although to be fair, my mum had started to teach me piano at home aged 6. Jill Bowman taught me viola from an equally early age and I am now toying with the idea of picking up again where I left off – at the age age of 19. My background began with Classical Music, learning piano and viola at Terrington, whilst singing in the school choir every week. Then, at Durham this continued steadily, learning orchestral Viola, solo Piano, and singing in the school Choir as a Bass. There had been a 'Yorchestra' transitional youth music course in the summer holidays in between leaving Terrington and starting Durham. Guitar and Harmonica were interests that came to me later in life in my twenties.

It wasn't until I attended Hull University that more Popular and Jazz music began to appeal to me and make sense to play. If it wasn't for my mother making me practice for twenty minutes every day at an early age and rewarding me with a sweet after practice, I may never have developed a continuing interest in music the way I see it today. Piano was something that I hated – absolutely considered it foreign territory - for years. Not until

Grade 6 at Durham did I consciously realise I enjoyed playing. Likewise with viola and theory, as a child i hated studying these.

While attending Durham School I was drafted into the school Orchestra on viola. The main reason why Mr Jonathan Newell awarded me a music Exhibition to attend the school was the fact that I played viola. As the years progressed my interest grew and I would fantasise about playing a great concerto one day and being in a professional orchestra. When Mr Roger Muttitt took over as Music Director he organised a massive concert where he conducted Elgar's Dream of Gerontius in York Minster. There were hundred's of singers and orchestral members – I was a singer (Bass). Half-way through the concert his baton flew out of his hand into the audience – funny!

My friend Chris Cartner was organ scholar in the school chapel, and oboist/pianist/conductor, too. He had some magnificent recordings of the Beethoven symphonies by the Berlin Philharmonic Orchestra, conducted by Herbert Von Karajan. We used to joke with each other about playing for them one day – of course that day never came about. I struggled to keep up with the Northern Junior Philharmonic Orchestra, and Newcastle's Young Sinfonia. For both of these I had 'hacked' through the audition on my viola, but owing to the need for viola players I was offered a place. The NJPO gave a huge concert in Ripon cathedral at the 1996 International Ripon Festival. We played an assortment of music, including Stravinsky's Firebird, and Michael Tippett's Shire Suite and The Rose Lake. The Young Sinfonia rehearsed every Sunday in Newcastle and gave concerts every season, including touring on the continent. I was with them for one year. Our repertoire included Mendelssohn's Hebrides Ouverture, Beethoven's Romance, and a Mozart Symphony.

Also, in the school holidays, I attended Xenophon Kelsey's Dales Chamber Orchestral holidays on viola. We played works including Wagner's Siegfried Idyll and I attended several courses there before I lost interest, aged 19, in December 1997. Suddenly all that I had aspired towards as a teenager was no longer appealing to me – now that I could have realised what I had tried to do for so long. That was the last time I actually played viola as a part of something good. I can recall sharing some cannabis on an evening with other musicians. It seemed like a bohemian and an artistic thing to do at the time.

In terms of exam standards, I ended up with Grade 5 Singing, Grade 5 Theory, Grade 7 Viola, and Grade 8 Piano. All ABRSM exams. It wasn't supposed to end there, but my Mental Health had something to do with that. Today, I still dream of furthering my musical repertoire and standard, therefore considering diplomas, further grades, and learning guitar and harmonica. Aged 17, I had a grand design to play jazz piano in a piano bar. It wasn't until 2009 – aged 30, that I achieved this goal, playing in the Whitby Marine Bar for family and general listening, and combining Thelonius Monk, George Shearing, Duke Ellington, Dave Brubeck, Antonio Carlos Jobim, Madeleine Dring, and a selection of popular hits. For me it was a dream come true, even though I don't think anybody else realised this about the occasion.

Over the years, my private recorded music collection increased as I bought and received CD's. My top ten albums, songs, and artists will be looked at in a moment. Also, public concert-going was something I enjoyed, ranging from musical shows/operas such as West Side Story (York), Joseph (Durham), Godspell (Durham), Mama Mia (London and Toronto), Our House (London), Les Miserables (London), South Pacific (York), The Magic Flute (Hovingham), The Marriage of Figaro (Hovingham), Gianni Schicchi (Helmsley), Falstaff (Leeds), and Don Carlos (Leeds). I was always with friends or family when attending a concert, caught up in the magic of music – lost in music!

Scarborough Acoustic Gathering in Peasholm Park, 2007-10, was a free event that I discovered whilst living in Scarborough. I attended three years running and enjoyed the lakeside performances there, mainly Guitar/Vocals. There were always others whom I knew there when I turned up!

On piano, while living in Scarborough, I had appearances in the annual Saltburn Music Festival as mentioned, Helmsley Art Centre Acoustic Night (where I had once been offered £15 for bar-jazz in 1998) and sang Roland Orzabal's Mad World and John Hiatt's Have a Little Faith in Me, and Scarborough: Westborough Church combining classical Mozart, Satie, Joplin, Jazz – Autumn Leaves, Pink Minor, Girl from Ipanema, Take Five, and Popular Ain't no Sunshine when she's gone; and the Grand Hotel similarly playing classical, jazz and popular – eg Round Midnight, Satin Doll, That Ole Devil Called Love, Elvis Costello's She, Elton John's Song for Guy, The Wasteland, Your Song, Sorry Seems To Be The Hardest Word, Lou Reed's Perfect Day, John Legend's Ordinary people, Alicia Keye's If I Ain't Got You, plus many more. At Saltburn my first programme involved a Haydn Sonata in Em, Bartok, Madeleine Dring, C P E Bach, and Scott Joplin. The second year included Mozart's Sonata in F, Chopin's Polonaise, Sinding's Rustle of Spring, Debussy's Clair de Lune, and another Scott Joplin Rag. And this year the programme includes Beethovens Sonata in Cm (Pathétique), Debussy Suite pour le piano, Bartok 6 Bulgarian Dances, and Gershwin's The Man I love and I Got Rhythm.

Chris Wright took me on as a piano student in August 2010, since which time we have been steadily working towards a classical piano diploma and some advanced theory, too.

The Jazz Festival I attended in Canada went East from Calgary, to Montreal, Quebec, and Ottawa. Whilst there on exchange year I sang three old songs over piano for an audience – Elton John's Your Song, The Hollies He Ain't Heavy He's My Brother, and John Lennon's Imagine, accompanied by Mario who played guitar and sang too. Scarborough's Jazz festival at the Spa saw me and David Ives attending two years running. I read in the Independent Newspaper about the Brussels, and Paris Jazz scene. I would love to go there in person one day. I love the thought of jazz on the streets and in the clubs and bars.

Moving on to my top twelve albums, artists (male and female), and songs. I have over 200 CD's in my collection ranging through Classical, World, Indie, Jazz, Dance/Trance, Latin, Ambient, Rock, Pop and Soul. From my collection I would select the following Albums as most listened to (in alphabetical order):

Male
Bryan Adams The Best Of Me
Coldplay Viva La Vida, Parachutes, & Rush of Blood to the Head Elton John Songs From The West Coast
Guns N' Roses Use Your Illusion I & II
James Blunt Back To Bedlam
Jamie Cullum Twenty Something
Jools Holland Jazz Piano
Radiohead OK Computer
Robbie Williams Live at Knebworth
Seal Soul
Simply Red Greatest Hits
The Best Power Ballads In The World

Female
Adele 19
Alicia Keys The Diary of Alicia Keys
Alison Moyet The Essential
Avril Lavigne Let Go
Carole King Natural Woman
Enya Paint the Sky With Stars
Leona Lewis Spirit
Madonna Ray Of Light
Marta Deyanova Mozart piano sonatas
Pink Missundaztood, Just Like a Pill
Texas White On Blonde
Saint Etienne Too Young to Die

Likewise, the following artists and songs are my personal favourites from over the years. Here are my top 15 most listened to songs in alphabetical order:

The Green Dragon

Male
Bruce Hornsby The Show Goes On
Chicane Offshore
Elvis Costello Oliver's Army, Alison, What's so funny bout-
Eric Clapton My Father's Eyes
Faithless Don't Leave
Khaled Aicha
Jackson Browne The Load Out and Stay
Jason Mraz Song for a Friend
KLF Justified and Ancient
Lionel Ritchie Hello, Stuck on you, Easy
Massive Attack Unfinished Sympathy
Michael Jackson We are the World
Moby Porcelain
TOTO Africa
U2 Still Haven't Found What I'm Looking For

Female
Annie Lennox Why
Bjork Play Dead
Carly Simon Baby you're the Best
Dido White Flag
Dido & DJ Tiesto You Take my breath away
Dionne Warwick & Stevie Wonder That's what friends are for
Gloria Estafan Rhythm's Gonna Get You
Gloria Gaynor I Will Survive
Kate Bush Man With the Child In His Eyes
Katrina Walking on Sunshine
K T Tunstall Suddenly I see
Lamb My Angel Gabriel
Sade No Ordinary Love
Sophie B Hawkins Damn I wish I was your lover
Taylor Dane Tell it to my heart

In July 2010, Mum and I went to see the Opera North Orchestra accompany Dame Kiri Te Kanawa, and Jose Carreras at Scarborough's Open Air Theatre. A year later, in June 2011,

Dave Ives and I went to see Elton John perform Live at the Open Air Theatre. And in between times, a few concerts at The Sage, Gateshead, with Dave and Alex; eg the Labeque sisters on piano (French-Canadians), Martin Taylor on guitar, the Hallé Orchestra conducted by Sir Mark Elder – Prokofiev's Piano Concerto, Elgar's Enigma Variations, Sibelius En Saga, and Dvoraks Slavonic Dances. Also, several operas at Leeds Opera North eg Don Carlos and Falstaff.

Next follows my CV:~

Jamie Kershaw - Curriculum Vitae

Gender: Male
DOB: 27/09/1978
Age: 32
Nationality: British

Work Experience:
- January and March 2010 ~ Piano Guest, Scarborough Grand Hotel
- October 2009 ~ Piano Guest, Scarborough Westborough Church (Charitable, Biographical Exhibition Event)
- September 2009 ~ Piano Artist, Helmsley Arts Centre 'Acoustic Night'
- August 2009 ~ Piano Guest, Whitby 'Marine' Piano Bar
- June 2009 & 2010 ~ Piano Artist at Saltburn Music Festival
- November 2008 ~ Piano Guest, Scarborough Library

(NB All the above for experience only)
- July/ August 2007 ~ *Rethink*, London – Interview technique (PT)
- September 2005-May 2006 ~ University of Hull *Student Facilitator/Healthy Volunteer* Participating in the development and training of Students (PT).
- September 2005- January 2006 Ramada Hull, Willerby, Hull – *Bar Staff/Waiter* Serving food and drink to guests, maintaining hygiene in the kitchen and bar areas. Handling finances reliably (PT).
- July/August 2004 – *Executive Officer:* The Pension Service, Stockton, Teeside, UK Research and compiling a key report for the government - Summer placement.
- July/August 2003 1)*Wine promotion assistant* : Kenwood House, London, UK

Preparing wine samples for potential customers at outdoor summer concerts.

2) Carpenter's assistant: London, UK. Assisting in various renovation projects - preparations, shelving, sanding, painting (PT).

- March – July 2001 Flamingo Land Theme Park and Zoo, Kirby Misperton, Malton, N Yorks, UK - *Bar staff, Catering, Amusements, Ride Operator & Ideas* Providing quality advice, service and guidance for visitors whilst maintaining a professional level of hospitality (FT).
- 09/2000-03/2001 - *Bar staff* Bright Steels Social Club, Wood Street, Norton/Malton, N Yorks, UK Participating in good customer relations whilst providing beverages and collecting glasses (PT).
- 09/1999-01/2000 – BATA Garage forecourt attendant Bondgate, Helmsley, N Yorks – friendly customer service with attention to detail.

Education & qualifications:
- July 2008 Spanish Intermediate ~ Foundation award
- November 2007 Craft of Script Writing for Film and TV ~ Foundation award (10 credits)
- 09/2002 - 06/2006 Hull University BA/Management (International) 2:2 Modules included: Human Resource Management, Marketing, Accounting, Entrepreneurship, Business Ethics, Strategic Management, Organisational Learning, Market Research.
- 09/2004 – 06/2005 exchange year at Dalhousie University, Nova Scotia, Canada. Modules included: Marketing Communications, Logistics Management, Organizational Change, International Business, New Venture Creation.
- November 2007 Anthony Robbins ~ Wealth Mastery Seminar, Ibis Hotel, Earls Court, London
- June 2007 Anthony Robbins ~ Unleash The Power Within (UPW): The Firewalk Seminar (Excel Centre, London Docklands, UK) & February 2006
- 2002 European Computer Driving Licence (ECDL) ~ Powerpoint, Databases, Spreadsheets, Word and Internet Communications
- 1997 Grade 8 Piano (Distinction), 1996 Grade 7 Viola (Merit), Grade 5 Singing and Theory (Pass)
- 09/1992 - 07/1997 Durham School, Durham City, UK

4 A-levels : Biology (B), French (C), Music (C), General Studies (B)
10 GCSEs @ A-C including English and Mathematics

Other achievements:
- 2010 Fiction Novel 'Plan 103f' published by www.chipmunkapublishing.com (first book)
- 2010 Autobiography completed 'The Green Dragon'
- April 2006 Paris Marathon (3:25)– raised £1,000 Get Kids Going!, ½ marathons Bath - March 06 (1:30), Bridlington Nov 05 (1:46), Great North Run Oct 02 (2:12) – raised £500 Cancer Research
- January 2006 IBM Universities Challenge Semi-Finalist (Procter & Gamble, Newcastle, UK) Test of initiatives, group dynamics, and creative powers
- February 2006 Basic Child Protection and Behaviour Management workshop
- October 2005 Royal Navy Leadership Development Course
- 2002-2004 St John Ambulance Basic First Aid skills (ECS, FAW, AED et al)
- 2000 Duke of Edinburgh Open Gold Award (North York Moors and Brecon Beacons, Wales; Voluntary work for Help The Aged and the less able)
- 1997 Full, Clean Driving Licence (Malton, N Yorks)

Other
Interests: languages (listening, speaking, reading and writing - Spanish intermediate, French A-level, Russian beginner), catering and cuisine, plus travel experiences European and Canadian.

References: available on request

Finally, the letter to Rethink upon moving out:~

Tuesday, 12th May 2009
Dear Rethink,

Though there are many of you, it is to all of you to whom I am writing. Really, I would like to say a very big thankyou for a wonderful two years at 6 Sussex Court. It is thanks to yourselves that this was even possible in the first place as my 'next step'.

As far as I can remember I would like to thank Joan, Stacy, Lesley, Ben, Lauren, Alison and Scarlett for spending some quality and productive time with me over this period. I handed the keys back to Yorkshire Coast Homes on Tuesday, 5th May. I am now happy with my new situation and forthcoming parenthood. It seems amazing that in a two year timeframe we have been through everything from jigsaw puzzling to local café culture, to a job in London, to goal setting and book writing, to dog ownership and then meeting Christina. As yet I am awaiting replies from 12 publishers/agents and have had three constructive rejections.

I have always had the notion that life is like a river – beginning small and remote, quietly trickling along, then gradually the water changes course, growing, meandering, deepening and running faster over rocks in places, never an easy journey but if you stick with it life can be rewarding in places, and that makes it all worthwhile! The river water always ends up out at sea or in a lake where we, as humans, have to learn to interact. Sometimes I wonder, wouldn't it be great to go back to the source and start all over again.

To begin with, in 2006-07 I would rather have remained an athlete, but by now I have adapted to other priorities and look forward to sharing more music with those who wish to listen. There is a lot more to say to you all than a single page letter, but

The Green Dragon

I hope that you will accept this simple note as a word of gratitude for all that you have done for me and continue to do for everyone at Rethink. I trust that the next tenant of Flat 6 will similarly enjoy their two years in a great home. This was the finest accommodation I have ever lived in, more so as in a ten year period I have lived in no less than 15 properties for between two months and two years each!

Thankyou once again, thanks a million!

Kind regards,

Jamie Kershaw (BA)

Appendices

The following ten pieces of work were written during my time at Hull University, and in my opinion these are my best ten pieces of written work, written between September 2002-May 2006. They are presented in chronological order, beginning with the earliest then working to the final year pieces. The index details their content.

The Green Dragon

Appendix 1 Human Resource Management (13/12/02: 12 pages)
Describe what Recruitment and Selection is and explain how it forms part of the human resource planning system within an organization. Also explain why these two processes are essential to good HR practice?

Appendix 2 The Management Process (19/12/03: 12 pages)
Why is language so central to organisational culture and how is this manifested in organisations?

Appendix 3 European Business (15/01/04: 13 pages)
Q 2)   Briefly outline the general basic mechanisms of the Single European Market. What has been the impact of the SEM on the airline sector?

Appendix 4 Marketing Information and Research (01/03/04: 11 pages) Marketing Analysis for Hull FC

Appendix 5 Research Methods (02/04/04: 14 pages)
Piracy and its effects on record sales in the Music Industry

Appendix 6 Understanding Organisation (30/04/04: 12 pages)
Compare and contrast the approach of any three paradigms to the role of management theory and practice. Chosen paradigms are: Interpretivism, Functionalism, and Critical Theory.

Appendix 7 Logistics Management (22/01/05: 11 pages)

Appendix 8 Business Development and the Entrepreneur (21/10/05: 17 pages) **Q2)**   Evaluate the net economic benefits that two specific mainland European regions have received, during this decade, from UK and Eire basedlow-cost airlines establishing continental European-based operational bases. These regions will be in European countries such as France and Belgium, where EasyJet and Ryanair respectively have established routes to and from the UK and Eire.

Appendix 9 Strategic Management (23/02/06: 12 pages)

"Stakeholders are those individuals or groups who depend on the organisation to fulfil their own goals and on whom, in turn, the organisation depends". (Johnson & Scholes p179)

Using examples where appropriate, discuss how the strategy of an organisation might be affected if/when stakeholders pursue their own objectives.

Appendix 10 Independent Study (28/03/06: 25 pages)
Quasar Coffee Shop New Venture Creation

Appendix 1

Describe what Recruitment and Selection is and explain how it forms part of the human resource planning system within an organization. Also explain why these two processes are essential to good HR practice?

Human Resource Management
Assignment for 13/12/02

So, what is Recruitment and Selection? In the simplest of terms it could be described as being the process of choosing new staff to work for the organization. Recruitment being the actual acceptance and enrolling of the new employee(s), and Selection being the practice of choosing who is and who is not suitable or appropriate for working in any one particular company.

In terms of recruiting employees there are numerous factors which in total make up the recruitment process. The company in hand may be looking at points like the following three – 1) Who do we want working for us? 2) Getting the right people involved for the mutual benefit of both company and employees; and 3) The overall cost involved has to be accounted for. In other words the organization is responsible for defining the job to be done, defining the characteristics of the ideal candidate, attracting candidates and ultimately selecting the most appropriate candidates for the job. Trying to 'knock square pegs into round holes' is not conducive to effective management. For example, the Accountancy company Price-Waterhouse and Coopers would not want an applicant whose skills would be more suited to being an agricultural farmer – it would not fit. So in more detail, the latter four responsibilities could read as following ………

Stage one – Job analysis would involve identifying the specific tasks needed in order to accomplish the job at hand. Also, there would be an examining of the hows, whens and whys tasks are performed. Necessarily, identification of the main duties and responsibilities of the job would go ahead. Finally the physical (geographical location of the organization), social (number of employees and how they interact), and financial (both incoming and outgoing costs of the organization) conditions of the job should be analysed.

Stage two – defining the characteristics of the ideal candidate. For this we could use Rodger's 'seven point plan' which describes the features that employers may look out for when recruiting candidates into their organization…

1) Physical appearance – looking out for recruits to be well dressed, have clear speech (articulate), and good health.
2) Attainments – scrutinizing the persons education, training , and work experience.
3) General intelligence – looking at the candidate to see if they are rational, logical, and have good analytical abilities.
4) Special aptitudes – checking recruits' oral and writing abilities.
5) Interests – for the recruit to say what they enjoy doing outside of the workplace.
6) Disposition – is the candidate acceptable, independent, and influential, or not?
7) Circumstances – somebody's personal life ie are they married with children? Also including an individual's travel quota in general. (Torrington, Hall & Taylor – HRM 5th edition – 2002 – p.191)

Stage three – attracting candidates to that particular organization. Here we look at advertising. In schools, colleges and universities the target group is slightly different for each of the three institutions, but nonetheless crucial in terms of potential recruits;

employment agencies (private and public) such as job centres where it is all computerised these days; casual callers on the telephone network trying to recruit individuals by chance; recommendations by other employers based on solid experience already had in the workplace; local and national newspapers contain adverts for positions of employment; local media – radio, television and magazines; head-hunting – attempting to obtain somebody already in employment elsewhere into a more senior position in another company ie your own; advertising on the Internet means that a larger circulation is attained because millions of people this day and age are on-line; Finally there are advertisements, both internal and external, in relation to the specific organization at hand.

Stage four – Selecting candidates for the organization. This will be looked at in more detail later on, but in brief, simple terms the employer undertakes practices such as shortlisting – in order to reduce the number of applicants down to a manageable size ; also there is a definite attentiveness towards seeking cost-effective employees, and finally there is the interview process which in itself often differentiates between acceptable and unacceptable candidates for recruitment. The interview process is a key factor of the selection process and shall be looked into later.

In addition to these four stages, the employer is still left with much more to do in terms of recruiting the most appropriate candidates. Work still to do would involve the following: assessing CV's (NB the equal opportunities policy overcoming discrimination), deciding which skills are essential and which skills are merely desirable, personal recommendations from previous contacts, knowing what the minimum requirements are for the organization involved. The list phases into the Selection methods which will also be dealt with later.

Firstly, assessing a Curriculum Vitae; A potential recruiter would want to see a well-structured and chronological application. It would be of value to assume a certain amount of creative editing on a CV to give the applicant a more favourable impression than is necessarily the case in reality. You may ask yourself is the candidate making a logical career choice by applying to your organization? Also there should be no gaps in the work experience sector, even if it includes periods of unemployment or sickness.

Secondly, choosing between desirable and essential skills. A restaurant eg pizza hut, would consider a different set of skills to be essential than would a professional football team eg Chelsea. The former would require as essential, skills as a pizza chef in order that the food is made as quality as is possible for the customers, and skills as a waiter ie promptness, good memory and good communication skills between themselves and the customers; also money-handling skills in order that the cash register be kept up to date and contain the correct information. It would be desirable for the fellow employees to get along but not essential to the job. The latter would require as essential physical fitness and agility in order that the players be on top of their game, ability to 'read' other players' moves at all times during the game in order that better physical positions on the pitch can be obtained for the game to flow smoothly. As for desirable skills it would again be desirable but non-essential for the players to get on with one another as people, but not essential to the game at hand.

Thirdly, looking at personal recommendations, one company might be more than willing to provide references for a fellow employee who is moving on to a new job, maybe with a better salary and higher up the ladder. For example, a school teacher of Geography may be offered a position as head of department – in another school – and consequently decide that they want to change to the better job offer. Their current colleagues may be more than willing to provide references to help them on their way. This is an example of a personal recommendation.

However there are problems recruiting in the wider market, and they include – how and where to advertise, how to determine a level of pay, how to assess the technical skills and abilities of candidates NB different countries have very different styles of education and training, and how to assess the willingness of the candidate to adapt to cultural norms of the recruiting organization. Common attributes that a multi-national company (such as HSBC, Barclays, McDonalds, Coca-Cola..) may look out for include: fluency in the English language, international experience, adaptability ie willingness to relocate throughout Europe, or indeed, the world.

There are two further reasons why Recruitment has become more difficult over the last decade through the 1990s. Firstly there is the problem that increasing numbers of potential recruits have been tempted to work abroad as growing awareness of the wider market in the international community came about. In addition to this there has been a downturn of school leavers and qualified graduates entering the labour market, which has previously been the main target for recruiters. Many employers in Britain have lost their professional staff to Europe and beyond and will remain to do so unless they rethink their policies on recruitment and retention.

However, continuing in this vein, there are problems encountered in reality which even the most prepared of HR teams has to deal with, such as accidents happening at work resulting in somebody going to hospital for treatment, a period of low productivity from the workforce; also there is a chance that somebody may have very few, or low, versatility skills and consequently find it hard to adapt to new technology and changing methods within the workplace regardless of what their cv claimed.

This concludes the section on what is recruitment and some of the potential downfalls of the process. Now we shall look at the *selection* aspect. It is very much a two-way process with the influence passing between selector and candidate. The interview enables the interviewer to discover which of the candidates live up to expectations and who best meets the job's requirements. The interview enables the interviewee to find out about the job and the organisation; also it is chance to decide if they really want to work for you. Whether successful or rejected the candidate should leave the interview with a favourable impression of the company and feel none the worse about themselves as a result of the interview. The manager feels their own authority by being in the position of employer/interviewer and the candidate has the right to ask questions of the interviewer also. Both employer and potential employee make decisions throughout the course of the selection procedure.

Similar to Rodger's seven point plan, but equally relevant to the selection process is Fraser's fivefold grading:

1) Impact of individual on others - are they influential?
2) Qualifications or acquired knowledge – gained at school, college or university.
3) Innate abilities – natural skills such as communication ability, body language etc
4) Motivation – willingness to get on with the job at hand.
5) Adjustment or emotional balance – are they a stable person or are they neurotic?
(Torrington, Hall & Taylor – HRM 5th edition – 2002 – p.191)

However, the selection procedure proves to be often unreliable, invalid and subjective. The following four reasons look into the interview procedure:

1) First impressions are often formed within the first three to four minutes of an interview and the remainder of the time is spent on proving that first impression to be right.

2) Sometimes candidates arrive at an interview and the selector is unwilling to change their opinion formed from reading their cv and the candidates first appearance.

3) There is more weight balanced on any unfavourable evidence/information than that on the favourable side.

4) Once an interviewer has made up their mind about an interviewee their behaviour could start to betray the candidate.
(Webster – 1964)

Whereas in an effective HR plan, detailed recruitment and selection procedures would be practised, a badly organised HR plan would result in a mess and everybody would become confused and disenchanted because of the lack of organization. So where there is bad HR planning it could be likened to old wine in new bottles – initially seeming ok but quickly loses its appeal once the curtains have been undrawn.

As the interview procedure is a central feature of the Recruitment and Selection process it can be seen to be often a biased event due to the above four reasons. Let us look briefly at some **European schemes of selection**. For example, in France they have very diverse recruitment methods such as the use of minitel computer and the information network/super-highway aka the internet; also they hold recruitment fairs, have employment agencies (who target graduate-level recruits), use job advertisements and take note of personal recommendations. In Belgium there is a total dominance of Brussel's employment as their recruitment agencies are very highly developed. Holland consists of more flexible working practices in order to increase attractiveness of employers and to improve productivity. ie part-time work is seen as the way forwards in maintaining economic success. Spain enjoys a booming economy, or has done previously, due to diversification of its industry. Really the problem lays not in labour shortage but in skills ie finding the right person for the right job. Two major considerations relate to this section on Europeanism and selection. They are that first of all, the term 'European' or 'International' is often used to attract new recruits, and is not in itself real and meaningful. The term is merely a buzz word to attract attention. These companies are often no different from domestic organizations. Secondly it is important to recognise that forward-looking organisations take a lateral view and aim to recruit people who show promise of adapting to an international environment although not already operating at that level.

So, in order to improve working practice and efficiency there are three key points to take into account. Firstly, the employers must be flexible, the company's recruitment practices must be innovative, and links between companies and educational institutes must be enhanced. Secondly it is important that other countries take note of what each other is doing and how they operate eg Germany's liaison between school/employer, and France's diversity of graduate recruitment practices. Thirdly there is the equal opportunities policy (eg women on maternity leave wanting to return to employment after a certain amount of time; part-time workers being given their fair share of work; people not born as a native to the country in which they are making a job application). Selection becomes more arbitrary the closer it gets to making a firm decision, consequently people try to make a favourable impression of themselves. This is where application forms have their merit – forming a level grounding for all applicants. The transition between education and work is an area for careful management both by governments and employers.

Finally the reasons for the two processes being essential to good HR practice could read as follows...One of the very first events of becoming employed, or economically viable, is by means of the recruitment and selection process. This relates to Rodger's seven point plan and Fraser's five-fold grading as previously outlined. These key points will always feature where there is good HR planning.

In conclusion to this description and explanation it could be said that recruitment is the process of seeking new members to join an organization, selection is the process of choosing specifically who gets the job. In order that the new recruit(s) fit in, there ought to be a period of integration within the company. So, recruitment and selection form the preliminary impressions of an organization – that is from the point of view of employee as opposed to customer or consumer. An explanation why these two processes are essential to good HR practice could be that no organization would function effectively without a rigorous selection or interview process. It would not be practical to allow any Tom, Dick or Harry onto the workforce – the chances are that they would not possess the necessary skills needed in order to accomplish the tasks and jobs expected of them; an employee's level of skill has to match the employer's expectations, and this is decided as a result of the recruitment and selection procedure.

Bibliography

Albrow M (1997) *Do Organizations have feelings?* – Routledge - London

Attwood, Margaret (1989) *Personnel Management* – The Macmillan Press ltd –London – chapter 3

Heller R & Hindle T (1998) *Essential Manager's Manual* – Dorling Kindersley - London – pp.626-694 'Interviewing people'

Hesselbein F, Goldsmith M & Beckhard R (1997) *The Organization of the future* - Jossey Bass Publishers - San Francisco

Martin J (2001) *Organizational Behaviour 2nd edition* – Thomson learning – Italy – p.152

Pinder M (1990) *Personnel management for the single European market* – Pitman publishing – London

Rowntree D (1996) *Manager's book of checklists* – Pearson Education ltd – Bolton

Torrington D, Hall L & Taylor S (2002) *Human Resource Management 5th edition* – Prentice Hall – chapters 11 and 12

http://www.google.co.uk "Human Resource Management recruitment and selection"

http://www.hull.ac.uk/lib/eir/athens.htm "HRM recruitment and selection

Appendix 2 - Why is language so central to organisational culture and how is this manifested in organisations?

Language *is* central to organisational culture. Here we shall look into varying aspects of both language and then culture, and how the one affects the other. The diversity of language will be explored relating specific examples of different organisations to their making use of different terminology. The importance of symbolism to culture will also be approached....using examples of organisations with their own unique symbols in order to establish an identity. It could be said that 'Culture is the invisible glue that holds an organisation together[1]'. Let us begin with some definitions.....

Language is the method of human communication, either spoken or written, consisting of the use of words in an agreed way[2]. In the form of codes, symbols, anecdotes and rules about appropriate statements, language plays an important role in organisational culture, constituting a large part of the shared understanding held by the organisation's members[3].

Culture is that complex whole which includes knowledge, belief, art, morals, law, custom and any other capabilities and habits acquired by man as a member of society[4]. Culture is the system of meanings which are shared by members of a human grouping and which define what is good and bad, right and wrong and what are the appropriate ways for members of that group to think and behave. Culture creates *nomos* (order) out of chaos. *Nomos* is an area of meaning carved out of a vast mass of meaninglessness, a small clearing of lucidity in a formless dark, always ominous jungle.[5]

Firstly, language has many intricacies and idiosyncrasies to deal with. Let us look at a few which may crop up within an organisation like ZTC Ryland.....there is the *mnemonic* 'POSDCORB'[6] used by management. It stands for Planning, Organising, Staffing, Directing, Co-ordinating, Reporting, and Budgeting. This mnemonic was created ensure that values are shared equally by all employees and clients/customers too. Let us also look at the following.....*Anaphora* – the repetition of first words in each new sentence – eg 'You know what the business requires of you. You know what's in it for you. You know that in the end you've got to persuade yourself'. *Personification* –

---

[1] Journal of General Management (vol 28 no 1 Autumn 2002: p.16)
[2] Oxford English Reference Dictionary (1996 : p.804)
[3] Management Science Journal (vol 49 no 4 April 2003: p.402)
[4] Hatch M J (1997: p203) Organization Theory
[5] Watson T J (2001: pp21/22) In search of Management
[6] Watson T J (2001: p35)

The Green Dragon

treating the business as if it were a living entity with needs eg 'You know the way the business needs to go'. *Simile*: 'it's like making an investment'; and *metaphor*: ' his mistake was glaringly obvious'[7]. In addition to these examples, language makes use of *Morphemes* (the form of words), *Phonemes* (units of sound within words), and *Sememes* (units of meaning in a sentence or a phrase)[8]. These examples are just the tip of the iceberg. Here we are trying to relate how language manifests itself in culture and how the two interact.

Schein coined the term 'psychological contract'[9] and is related to how employees express their dedication and commitment to the organisation and is also relevant to ensuring that employees regularly meet expectations along the way. A psychological contract creates the opportunity for an employee to fulfil their personal values. Geertz decided that 'men spin webs of significance'[10] in order to feel fulfilled by going about their every day business. People like to feel important. The concept of *simultaneous tight-loose controls* within an organization is important as it toys with the psychological contract of choosing to work because you want to, not because you have to.[11]

There are different forms of verbal communication…dialogue and rhetoric. Walter Nash defines rhetoric as being "an ordinary human competence…..an ordinary thing with some extraordinary manifestations, some graceful, some less so"[12].

Let us now look at how different organisations portray their differences. Language is one factor….. by means of idiosyncrasies and unique phrases to that particular organisation these differences are portrayed. For example at Air Traffic Control the terminology would not be the same as at a Telephone

---

[7] Watson T J (2001: p.185) In search of management
[8] Landar H (1966: p.53) Language and Culture
[9] Watson T J (2001: pp 61-63)
[10] Hatch M J (1997: p.218) Organization Theory
[11] Watson T J (2001: p.16)
[12] Watson T J (2001: p.183)

Call Centre. In the first instance one may hear phrases such as "You may now taxi to the runway", or "You are clear to land", whereas at a call centre they may use language such as "Please continue to hold, the operator knows you are waiting......., ...your call is very important to us, thankyou for continuing to hold". Likewise there would be differences between Movie Direction and the Military. In the organisation of movie-making, language such as "Action! – Cut!", or "That's a rap!" would be frequently used by the Director. In the Military one would often hear "Attention!", or "Stand at ease!", especially whilst on parade in the army. In organisations today you may hear or say certain buzz words and phrases such as 'we strive towards interdependence', 'let's synergise', 'together we should be proactive', or 'think win/win'. Phrases such as 'a quitter never wins and a winner never quits' ought to boost morale. There are also many other examples of organisations in which the management would use different terminology in order to be meaningful to that particular set of people in that particular situation.

Secondly there is culture ..... there is <u>official culture</u> – 'the system of meanings, values and norms espoused by the managerial dominant coalition', and there is <u>unofficial culture</u> – 'systems of meanings, values and norms actually prevailing in the organisation'[13]. It is all about taking the rough with the smooth, life is not all a bed of roses, there are Guns and there are roses. In moments of difficulty such as being "up shit creek without a strategy/paddle", ZTC Ryland insists on their 'strategic intent', 'winning culture', and 'DOC' initiatives (which will be examined later) to remain focused on their goals and to keep a customer focus. A manager may be heard to say "get back to the knitting" in order to keep everybody's feet on the ground and heads out of the clouds. ZTC has been compared to a heroic Shakespearean character 'vaulting ambition, which o'er leaps itself'[14] in the sense that it has set a target to quadruple the annual turnover in a relatively short space of time. ZTC Ryland

---

[13] Watson T J (2001: p.112)
[14] Watson T J (2001: p.157)

has very much bitten the bullet in setting such a high target. All this and all the time contending with Murphy's law – if anything can go wrong it will go wrong – but the positive initiatives are all in place therefore the company stands a strong chance of achieving its aims.

Culture is a survival mechanism which may be more narrowly or more broadly adaptive, and which may obstruct or facilitate the survival of the organism as it singles it out from or integrates it into a wider group[15]. Culture controls behaviour and there are frequent battles between Democracy and Bureaucracy, Ideology and Hegemony, and individuals with divergent interests where unity is required[16].

Organisations come in many different shapes and sizes, from religious or educational organisations to profit making multi-national corporations as is the example of ZTC Ryland. There are many cultural influences in society eg family, community, nation, state, church, education and business organizations. These shape attitude, behaviour and identity[17].

Thirdly, Symbols are a major part of organisations. With symbols we can identify what is what in our social culture. Awareness of culture is not enough in itself – we have to act and change with the times as culture is always changing just as surely as the world keeps on spinning[18].

Society learns to associate establishments with symbols. For example, in religion where the church is the organisation, there is the Bible, and a Biblical principle that everyone ought to live by in business and life is: "people will do what you require of them if you treat them as you would want to be treated yourself"[19].

---

[15] McQuown N Language, Culture and Education (1982: p.46)
[16] Hatch M J (1997: pp 327-349)
[17] Hatch M J (1997: pp200-236)
[18] Clark H, Chandler J & Barry J (1994: pp373-381) Organisation and Identities
[19] Watson T J (2001: p.170)

There are different texts for different religions eg Muslims use the Koran, Hindus read the Bhagavadgita, and Christians read the Bible, and people do live by these books. In the UK in today's society there is a lot of open-mindedness when it comes to religion. Hence the modernization of serious religious events in the form of musicals, such as Godspell, Jesus Christ Superstar and the Last Temptation of Christ, is no longer controversial. In times gone by these musicals would have caused an absolute outrage, but today we appreciate such works. Today's society is comparatively free-thinking.

In Victorian times when the church was in a highly authoritative state of existence, many people were reprimanded for certain linguistic breaches. One such case was a writer, Mr Moxon who wrote: "they have three words: well tyrants know their use, well pay them for the loan, with usury torn from a bleeding world. God, Hell, and Heaven......" he was punished for insinuating that God, Hell, and Heaven are merely words[20]. How times have changed!

Symbols of Educational organisations are also prominent. For example here at Hull University there are five representative symbols. They are the Kingston-upon-Hull crown, the dove of peace, the torch of learning, the white rose of Yorkshire, and the fleur-de-lis of Lincolnshire. These symbols have been chosen to symbolise the educational organisation which is Hull University.

In Russia a very important term for the people is that of *Perestroika*.....the restructuring of the entire political and economical system advocated by the then President Mikhail Gorbachev throughout the 1980s. Used in conjunction with the term *Glasnost,* the then USSR altered and gained greater awareness of economic markets worldwide, moved away from central planning, learnt greater tolerance for religious worship,

---

[20] Marsh J (1998: p.91) Word Crimes

opened up to more reporting of events in the USSR and globally, and offered rehabilitation to dissidents[21].

ZTC Ryland is symbolised by '1+2+3+4=5'. There is more to this than numbers alone; acting as part of the organisation's mission statement, this represents first-place in Britain, second in Europe, third in the US, and fourth in the Far East. Their intention is to be ranked fifth among telecommunications worldwide. Currently a £1.28 Billion company, the goal is to become a £5 Billion company within six years. This enormous aim requires very positive steps to be taken and ZTC Ryland have devised a set of slogans to enforce the 'winning culture' ideal within the organisation. These slogans are as follows[22]:

- Bringing people together
- Responsive to customers
- Commitment to excellence
- Recognition of individual contribution
- Willingness to change
- Profitability, technology, growth

Employees may think of the above as just being flavours of the month and temporary, but the intention is to put words into practice and walk the talk. The saying "a rose by any other name would smell as sweet"[23] means that it would still be the same organisation regardless of the symbols chosen to represent it. ZTC Ryland is the result of a merger between Parry and ZEC. Their objective is to create one new culture to replace two old cultures- not to merely takeover aimlessly! In order to help this process, ZTC have developed a programme called Developing Organisational Capabilities (DOC) with a slogan of "working through people". Along with their 'strategic intent' and 'winning culture' goals DOC is designed to create the new culture. What was originally the 'Business Improvement

---

[21] Ries N(1997) Russian Talk – culture and conversation during Perestroika

[22] Watson T J (2001: pp95/96)

[23] Landar H (1966: p.51) Language and Culture

Programme' (BIP) became the 'Personal Development Programme' (PDP) – note the use of acronyms demonstrating a connection between language and culture – created to dispense shared values amongst employees. Two other Total Quality Management (TQM) initiatives put to use at ZTC Ryland are the 'Business Action Teams' (BATs) each tackling a specific problem, and these would be co-ordinated by the 'Business Improvement Teams' (BITs) who would cover broad areas like production, personnel, or purchasing. One manager described these initiatives of being "more fads with fancy names", thus expressing their doubt about the scheme's effectiveness[24].

Culture is there to describe and explain social phenomena. Also, culture is to be manipulated in order to improve performance, hence the need for ZTC Ryland to use the 'winning culture' slogans – to manipulate the employees who form part of the organisational culture. Shared values formulate society's culture, and values change over time, being reflected in language, working arrangements and styles.[25] British Telecom (another telecommunications giant) has been committed to Total Quality Management since 1986, as a way of achieving its vision of being the world's top telecommunication's agency. BT uses values such as :

- Always put the customer first
- Ensure that there is mutual respect
- Demonstrate the importance of team-work
- Strive for continual improvement
- Act professionally (ie *walk the talk*)

We have looked at examples of how organisations differ and also how there is unity in diversity. One new aspect to consider is that in present day society the English language is commonly accepted as the main International language. This is not entirely without challenge. There is in existence a language invented

---

[24] Watson T J (2001: pp97-99) In search of Management
[25] Clark H, Chandler J & Barry J (1994: pp373-376) Organisation and Identities

over 100 years ago; the language is completely International with millions of speakers the whole world over. It is called *Esperanto*. There are no known cultural barriers for this language and it also has its own literature. It would take a Global Revolution, but this language could be the answer to many a problem eg in an organisation such as the United Nations, important meetings could be conducted in Esperanto rather than requiring many translators for all the different languages. This would cut costs enormously and make huge International savings. Were Esperanto to be fully-supported and taught in schools, colleges and universities throughout the international community this would be a major solution to many difficulties, saving £Millions.

Moving on, in *popular culture* today we are all subject to the media, music (of all genres), literature, sport, art, and movies at the cinema. We involve ourselves in the decision-making process of what is an average run-of-the-mill product, and what is a classic piece of art about to stand the test of time. By means of television popular culture is transmitted to the entire world. In music many bands have gone on to attain number one status for a song because it was played in a commercial and positive associations were made between the song and the product. For example *The Hollies* "He ain't heavy he's my brother" was played in a Miller Lite lager/beer advert and subsequently went on to become number one. Also *Ben E King's* "Stand by me" used in a Levi Jeans advert was a number one shortly after. *Luciano Pavarotti* shot to international fame after he sang 'Nessun Dorma' – the theme tune for the 1990 World Cup football tournament[26]. There is an eternal battle between popular tabloid (eg The Sun, The Daily Mirror) newspapers and quality broadsheets (eg The Times, The Guardian). Everybody can identify with rock stars, detective heroes, football teams or religious/political leaders in some way[27].

---

[26] Storey J (1993: p.16) An introductory guide to cultural theory and popular culture
[27] Watson T J (2001: p.22)

William Shakespeare died just less than four hundred years ago, but his work is viewed today as the *epitome of high culture*. In his day people would have understood it as popular theatre possibly without realising the longevity of Shakespeare's genius.[28] Story-telling reinforces organisational culture. In popular culture we can all relate in some way to real life stories of war, murder, achievement and love transmitted through the media.[29]

Humour could be thought of to be a serious matter. For example an insult to an individual may be thought of as humour by the rest of the group eg "I wouldn't like to look like him for all the tea in China!", or to someone who is angry about an incident someone may ask "who's pissed in his chips?".[30]

And so, in conclusion it can be seen that language with all its subtleties and nuances is indefatigably central to organisational culture in many different ways. Good managers ensure that information and ideas are communicated clearly and unambiguously, with the appropriate choice of communication medium to maximise understanding on the part of the audience[31]. Language can be used to motivate, boost morale, unify, joke, share meaningful and progressive conversations, reprimand, discipline, instruct, create and many more options too. Language manifests itself in organisations by means of conversations, adverts, media attention eg breaking news, and internet information/emails. Organisations rely on dedicated and committed communicators to run the show by means of language and walking the talk.

(Word Count : 2575 words)

---

[28] Storey J (1993: p.8)
[29] Watson T J (2001: p.21)
[30] Watson T J (2001: pp162/187)
[31] Watson T J (2001: p.228)

Bibliography

Clark H, Chandler J, & Barry J (1994) *Organisation and Identities – text and readings in organisational behaviour* – Chapman and Hall – Oxford

Gleeson P & Wakefield N-eds(1968)*Language and Culture*–San Fran. State College

Hatch M J (1997) *Organizational Theory – Modern symbolic and postmodern perspectives* – Oxford University Press UK

http://proquest.umi.com/keyword 'Esperanto'

http://proquest.umi.com/keywords 'Language and culture'

Journal of Management Studies – Vol 40 No 4 June 2003 – Blackwell

Journal of General Management–Vol 28 No 1 Autumn 2002– The Braybrooke Pressltd

Landar H (1966) *Language and Culture* – Oxford University Press

Management Learning (Journal) – Vol 34 No 2 June 2003 – SAGE Publications

Management Science (Journal) – Vol 49 No 4 April 2003 – INFORMS

McQuown N (1982)*Language, Culture and Education*–Stanford Uni Press, California

Nauerby T (1996) *No Nation is an Island...Language, Culture and National Identity in the Faroe Islands* – North Atlantic Publications – Aarhus University Press

Ries N (1997) *Russian Talk – Culture and conversation during Perestroika* – Cornell University Press

Storey J (1993) *An introductory guide to Cultural Theory and Popular Culture* – Harvester Wheatsheaf

Turville P T (1996) *England the Nation* – Oxford University Press : New York

Watson T J (2001) *In Search of Management* - Thomson

Appendix 3 - Briefly outline the general basic mechanisms of the Single European Market. What has been the impact of the SEM on the airline sector?

The Single European Market (SEM) is an association of countries trading without restrictions, especially in the European Community. The EC is a major global superpower. Many of its companies are world leaders. In the 1980s the European Community was faced with a double crisis: loss of global economic competitiveness and the stagnation of political and economic integration[32]. Consequently a solution was required. The answer was to be the Single European Market. The SEM became established from 1st January 1993 as a result of the Single European Act (SEA), which by approved decree of the European Council came into force 1st July 1987. The SEA, in 1986, paved the way for the Single Market in 1993[33]. The creation of this huge common market has influenced major foreign investors to move into Europe.

The SEM exists to improve performance of European enterprises as a precursor to broader industrial success within international markets. The mechanisms of the SEM include lowering costs, thereby increasing competition and pushing up trade too. The idea being to create more growth and more jobs. The initial stimulus for the 1992 Single Market programme was Political rather than Economical. The SEA defined the internal market as: 'an area without internal frontiers in which the free movement of goods, persons, services and capital is ensured'[34]. There is a certain amount of spillover into other areas eg labour, energy, and the EMU. There is a constant need for new policies eg Trans-European Networks (TENS) to make the SEM work. This spillover is known as the 'snowball effect'.

Further benefits to enterprises' logistical chains are derived from the following issues:

---

[32] Williams (1995:91) The European Community
[33] The Oxford English Reference Dictionary (1996:1353)
[34] Williams (1995:91)

A) suppliers would lower there prices and raise the quality of products on offer.
B) production systems…the ongoing development of new locations to enter new markets and the lowering of the cost of market entry.
C) distribution systems…competition in services to the firm can further increase efficiencies NB transport, warehousing, and retailing[35].

All members were expected to gain in this exercise of deregulation.

There are even more insider advantages of the SEM…..there is a certain closeness to the market both geographically and commercially (marketing and manufacturing) whereby insiders gain better market information. Membership raises image and local identity, the aim being to establish 'local firms' with an understanding of local culture. Members have access to public procurement – non EU firms may only win contracts if they have a local market presence[36]. The EU provides stimulating demand for products and services.

The SEM programme seeks to unify the fragmented national markets into an integrated whole. The initial programme only had limited success in achieving its stated aims so it is very much an ongoing process. Also, the European Union has moved into the next phase of SEM development notably by extending its relevance and ensuring the full implementation of legislation. The Single European Market is coupled with greater openness to the global marketplace, both in terms of trade and also in terms of Foreign Direct Investment.[37]

Concerning the Internal Market strategy 2003-2006 there is a ten point plan to facilitate enlargement. The design is as follows:

---

[35] Johnson D & Turner C (2001:49) European Business
[36] Mercado, Welford & Prescott (2001:100) European Business
[37] Johnson D & Turner C (2001:63)

1) Enforcing the rules
2) Integrating services markets
3) Improve free movement of goods/services
4) Meeting the demographic challenge
5) Further opening of network services
6) Simplified regulatory environment
7) More open procurement
8) Improve conditions for business
9) Reduce tax obstacles
10) Provide better information and citizen's needs[38]

In 1985 *The White Paper* by Lord Cockfield identified nearly 300 barriers to be removed by 1992 in order to create a better European Union. These included physical, fiscal and technical barriers. *Physical* - the elimination of all frontier controls on the movement of goods, people and capital such as customs duties, passports and health checks. Also, frontier posts on national borders such as public security, immigration and drug controls. *Fiscal* – harmonization of VATs and other purchase taxes in the EC. There were two bands of VAT agreed…..standard rate = 14-20%, reduced rate = 5-9%. Also excise duties would be cut. *Technical* – absence of common standards, regulations, public procurement practices, differing laws and practices, and subsidies were to be altered accordingly. In addition to the above there would be a 10-24% reduction in airfares. Ever since the 1985 Cockfield White Paper on the single market and the 1986 Single European Act, progress towards economic and monetary union has gathered pace.[39]

The SEM is a process not an end in itself. It acts as a moving target and will exist when all tradable goods and services are freely traded. The SEM is not complete or perfect. An example being its effect on the airline sector NB budget airlines (which will be looked into later). The single market project did not magically come to an end in December 1992 - there has been a

---

[38] Johnson D (2003) Lecture notes week 5
[39] Williams A (1995:111) The European Community

continuing flow of internal market legislation since then, and still continues today.

The EU is the world's most successful in terms of integration. Integration occurs in phases. Phase one being custom's union (completed in 1968) removing tariffs. Phase two being the single market, beginning 1st January 1993, involving: making the rules more effective – proper enforcement and simplification of both EU and national laws. Dealing with key market distortions (related to tax). Removing sectoral obstacles to market integration – pinpoint barriers and prevent emergence of new impediments. Delivering a single market for the benefit of all citizens – sustaining and enhancing levels of employment, and offering increased levels of social protection; and Phase three being the economic and monetary union ie the single currency, the 'euro'[40].

Notable reports and future estimates of the SEM's results were to be made by Cecchini and Baldwin. Cecchini estimates that both barriers and costs would be reduced thus increasing overall efficiency and releasing a whole new flow of innovations. There would be eliminations of customs' delays and costs. Public markets would be exposed to competition, financial markets would be liberalised and integrated, but as a result of broader supply there would be side-effects. The Cecchini report of 1988 predicted the following gains from development of the SEM: an estimated 4.3-6.8% gain to the Community's GDP. There would be two million extra jobs created. There would be overall positive effects on inflation and fiscal balances. Baldwin estimates that greater capital stock would result in a greater percentage of investment made per year. He concludes that the gains from the internal market will be in the region of 3.5-9%, as opposed to the 2.5-7% predicted by Cecchini.[41]

In terms of external trade performance, the EU has moved from an external trade deficit in 1992 to a 19.21 Billion Euros trade

---

[40] Johnson D (2003) Lecture notes 'SEM'
[41] El-Agraa A M (2001:173-180) The European Union

surplus in merchandise goods in 1998[42]. The EU creates red-tape for businesses, the SEM removes this red tape. Any '*acquis communautaire*' countries must comply in order to join. Notably, any new countries could be perceived as a threat attacking the existing market.

The following are examples of the economic rationale for developing the SEM: Enhanced integration and factor allocation mean that there is an increase in intra-EU imports for both manufacturing and services. Changes in the nature and pattern of trade mean a move away from inter-state specialisation towards more harmonious industrial structures. Efficiency and competition effects are realised through restructuring of European industries. Employment, income and convergence as exemplified in Ireland, Spain, Portugal and Greece have a faster growth rate than the rest of the EU.[43]

However, the SEM does have its problems, and two examples are as follows.....
the SEM is caught in a scheme similar of 'Russian Dolls'. The single market is used as a device to tidy up omissions from the original Treaty of Rome. Notably macro-economic management is essential as an election-winning instrument for EC governments. Consequently some political parties in some member states are reluctant to relinquish their control over this. The 1992 programme could be said to be equally as much about politics as it is about economics. Also, an issue is that of *Eurosclerosis*. It is a problem to the EU in that the European Community is condemned to producing lower and intermediate technology goods as it was squeezed out of high-technology sectors by Japanese and US competition. So the pressure of competition is directly responsible for certain downfalls.[44]

Moving on, what is the impact of the SEM on the airline industry? April 1997 saw the completion of the European civil

---

[42] Mercado, Welford & Prescott (2001:99)
[43] Johnson D & Turner C (2001:51/52)
[44] Williams A (1995:94 & 115)

aviation market. It delivered three packages: 1987– reformed capacity sharing practices
- granted limited fifth-freedom rights
- flexible procedures for fare approval
- removed single designation provisions

1990 – extended liberalisation measures in the above

1992 – full fifth freedom and cabotage* rights.
- licensed EU operators have access to all international routes and can charge any fare they wish.[45]

*Cabotage being the transportation of goods or passengers wholly within the territory of one country by lorries, vessels or aircraft owned by nationals of another country.

Airlines are forming global strategic alliances to cope with new competitive pressures eg The Star Alliance, The Atlantic Excellence Alliance, Northwest Airlines, British Airways and American Airlines.[46]

Until the 1980s air travel in Europe operated under guidelines set out in the Chicago convention (1944) ie each state has sovereignty over its own airspace and provided for states to reach bilateral agreements concerning the provision of air services between them. For example Northern Ireland was served from Great Britain by British Airways. The Irish Republic operated Aer Lingus with the GB team in 1936. Aer Lingus also began services to Europe after World War Two[47].

The late 1980s saw the liberalization of EU transport. In June 1986 the average European airfare was three times more expensive than its US counterpart. The third package in 1992 saw that measures removed significant barriers to entry by setting common rules governing safety and financial requirements for new airlines. By 1997 the regulatory framework for the EU was similar to that for US aviation. Since

---

[45] Johnson D & Turner C (2001:181)
[46] Johnson D & Turner C (2001:183/184)
[47] Blacksell M & Williams A (1994:209) The European Challenge

January 1993 EU airlines have been able to fly between member states without restriction and within member states (other than their own) subject to some controls on fares and capacity. National restrictions on ticket prices were removed.

The European airline industry is still much oriented towards outdated national boundaries. Therefore poorer productivity, lower profitability and greater operating costs than US airlines. Budget airlines would not be possible without the SEM. Roots of obstacles lies in politics (state aids), and lack of capacity (congestion, air traffic control, slot allocation, inadequate infrastructure): "by unilaterally granting US carriers traffic rights to, from and within the EU while ensuring exclusively for their own carriers the right to fly from their territory to the US, these member states create serious discrimination and distortions of competition, thereby rendering EU rules ineffective" (Commissioner Kinnock)[48].

The US have bilateral deals extended to European airlines, also there are to be more US airlines to profitable hubs eg Heathrow. The EU vows to end restrictions, to include ownership limits, to open access for EU carriers to the internal US market, and total deregulation of EU-US aviation (excluding technical and safety measures)[49]. Consequences of all this are the opening of lucrative transatlantic trade to increase competition, placing budget airlines on trans-Atlantic routes, challenging US restrictions – eg public officials must travel on US airlines, higher subsidies on US airlines than in Europe, and limits on foreign ownership.

In June 2003 the Council of Ministers gives the European Community power to negotiate international airline agreements for the whole EU. In October 2003 the 'Open Skies' talks began between the EU and US. National carriers are subject to competition, NB Sabena was a casualty of this; a question to consider is will there be others too? Remaining problems

---

[48] Johnson D & Turner C (2001:182)
[49] Johnson D (2003) Lecture notes week 6

include airport congestion, and higher costs persisting in Europe because of air-traffic-control fragmentation; previously the state would aid national carriers.

Today, the world's largest commercial aircraft manufacturer (Boeing) is set to be overtaken by 'Airbus'. Boeing will build 280 aircraft this year, Airbus will build 300. There are differences in features too such as having a wider fuselage, electrical not mechanically fit controls, cockpits designed for use in more than one aircraft. Airship's A380 is set for its first flight in 2005. It will gain 35% more passengers than Boeing's B747, and the airfare will be 20% cheaper[50].

Issues surrounding aviation industry cutbacks include: financial health of customers, terrorism, war, recession and SARS. Budget flights in the US – Southwest, Frontier, AirTran, JetBlue – and in Europe – RyanAir and EasyJet – are picking up in passenger numbers. In 1986 RyanAir commenced services between Dublin and London (Luton) so price wars emerged as British Airways and Aer Lingus lowered their fares too. Capital Airlines and BA ceased to operate to Dublin. British Midland have also overtaken Capital Airlines. For a long time Aer Lingus and BA operated the Dublin to London route jointly. Note that deregulation poses the greatest challenge to the smaller airlines[51].

The 'Luxembourg Agreement' became effective in January 1988. This allows international carriers to pick up passengers at an intermediate stop in another community country (subject to certain restrictions eg fares, number of passengers carried, and which airports to be used). So in April 1992 Aer Lingus began operating services from Dublin to Amsterdam, Copenhagen, Paris and Zurich via Manchester[52].

---

[50] Fortune – vol 148 no 10 (Nov 10 2003) 'Airbus'
[51] Blacksell & Williams (1994:211)
[52] Blacksell M & Williams A (1994:210)

Scheduled airlines established in the European Economic Area have risen from 77 in 1992 to 139 in the year 2000. Nearly ten years after the effective liberalisation of the air transport sector, the results are beyond dispute. The airline sector is extremely fast-growing, dynamic and competitive. Several airlines have been taken over or ceased to trade as a result of competition. There has also been an emergence of low cost or 'no frills' airline offering simpler service, use of secondary airports, and competitive airfare prices. There are now more, and better-value, promotional tariffs as a result of competition. The number of air routes between different member states of the EU has risen by some 30% since 1993[53].

There are five European Low Cost Carrier (LCC) airlines. In the UK we have EasyJet, Go, and Buzz; Ireland have RyanAir; and Belgium have Virgin Express. The current market share of low cost airlines within Europe is 10%. Two of the above-mentioned airlines were established as ancillary services to their mainline parent companies. They are 'Buzz' with 'KLM' and 'Go' with 'British Airways'.

There are a set of air passenger rights for passenger's boarding these budget aircraft. The rights involve the staff: providing assistance for passengers facing delays, allowing telephone reservations to be held or cancelled without commitment or penalty within 24 hours, providing prompt refunds, providing assistance to passengers with reduced mobility and special needs, and finally meeting passengers' essential needs during long, onboard aircraft delays[54].

In conclusion, advantages gained from the Single European Market include:

- Market integration piecing together a fragmented Europe into one unified whole.

---

[53] http://europa.eu.int/comm/transport/air/rules/bilan_en.htm
[54] http://www.eca-cockpit.com/LCC/single.htm

- The removal of barriers to the transactions of goods, services, capital and labour.
- The airline sector is experiencing an explosion of competition, so prices are reduced and there are more flights to get you where you want to go.

Finally, the completion of the single market is the central *raison d'etre* of the EC[55].

---

[55] Craig P & De Burca G (2003:1170) EU Law

Bibliography

Blacksell M & Williams A (eds)(1994) *The European Challenge – Geography and development in the European Community* – Oxford University Press

Business Week – European edition July 7th 2003 – *'Delta's flight to self-service'*

Craig P & De Burca G (2003) *EU Law – Text, cases and materials* – O.U.P.

El-Agraa A M (2001) *The European Union – Economics and policies* 6th ed – FT Prentice Hall

El-Agraa A M (1994) *The economics of the European Community* 4th ed – Harvester Wheatsheaf

Fortune –vol 148 no 10 (November 10th 2003) *'Airbus'*

George S (1996) *Politics and policy in the European Union* 3rd ed – O.U.P. New York

http://news.bbc.co.uk/1/hi/business/1217429.stm

http://europa.eu.int/comm/transport/air/rules/bilan_en.htm

http://www.eca-cockpit.com/LCC/single.html

http://www.tutor2u.net/case_study_European_Airlines.pdf

Johnson D & Turner C (2001) *European Business – policy challenges for the new commercial environment* – Routledge London

Johnson D (2003) *Lecture notes on SEM* – week 5

Mercado, Welford & Prescott (2001) *European Business* 4th ed – FT Prentice Hall

Williams A (1995) *The European Community* 2nd ed – Blackwell, Oxford, UK

Appendix 4 - Marketing Analysis for Hull FC

In a nutshell: Hull FC is the organisation in hand and, as a market researcher, we are required to analyse the environment in which Hull FC operates by means of secondary data. Hull FC is in the competitive sport and entertainment market – sport for the players, coaches and referees, and entertainment for the fans and supporters.

There are two types of environment to take into account for this analysis; firstly the macro-environment (factors such as political, economical, sociological, technological, legal, geographical, demographical, and psychographical), and secondly the micro-environment (factors such as competitors – direct and indirect -, complementors, and customers). The data collected would need to be accurate, relevant to today's market place, unbiased, and meaningful.

The Macro-Environment

Politically there is a territorial battle going on between Hull FC and their closest rivals The Kingston Rovers. Such is the rivalry that the reaction produces more dynamic energy in Hull thus keeping both organisations/clubs alive and in the game. Hull FC in itself is not the only attraction which draws people to the games; there are other attractions, venues, and facets surrounding their games at home in Hull that draw the crowds. These will be looked into in detail as part of the micro-environment analysis – competitors and complementors.

Economically, Hull FC have to take into account many issues in order to ensure their club turns over sufficient to maintain standards and reputation too. Ticket prices range from £5/game junior, and £16/game adult, to season passes which range from £28 junior, to £252 best seats adult price in the west family stand. These are not the only prices however, there are different prices depending on which stand you support from. In order to try and get fans getting the best deal possible, Hull FC have teamed up with other local organisations such as 'The Deep' to obtain special offer discount prices for those who buy season passes. Hull FC have many sponsors including: The Deep, Corporate Travel International ltd., East Yorkshire Coaches, Hull City Council, Jones Electrical Supply co ltd, and Williamson's Solicitors. Cause and effect is in play; action and reaction......if one local club does well, others will also benefit as a direct result of their success. This will also be scrutinized in the micro-environment analysis.

Sociologically we have issues past, present and future to contend with. Sociology looks into attitudes, behaviour, beliefs, culture, ideas and motivations. In the past Hull FC (previously the 'Sharks') have had successes, winning Championship titles and maintaining their place in the Super-league, and clearly there is pressure from all around to keep the results coming. The Director of rugby, Shaun McRae, and others on the coaching team eg First Team Coach John Kear, and Fitness and Strength Co-ordinator Billy Mallinson, ensure that the highest standards are maintained in the club. Fans develop an emotional attachment to their team, some younger fans maybe with aspirations of their own to play for Hull FC one day, or to be a coach or part of the management team. Public Relations (PR) play a big role in sociological factors – advertising in the media, local newspapers/radio, word of mouth, flyers and posters all contribute to raising the public's awareness of Hull FC, thus maintaining a regular, loyal clientele who form the body of supporters for the club. Hull FC use lucky mascots for their games; for the forthcoming match versus Warrington Wolves 13 year old Joanne Railton has been selected. This can only enhance the public's perception of Hull FC as an organisation as it seeks to involve everybody in their mission, from young mascot, to aspiring players, through to elderly supporters.

Technologically, the KC stadium began as an idea, then a blueprint, then it was built and became solid reality with the help of labourers, mechanics, engineers, architects, patrons and sponsors, and many others too. Hull City Council own the KC stadium and the Stadium Management Company (SMC) possess a fifty year lease. The overall cost of the KC stadium was about £44million, and the project took fourteen months to complete. The KC Stadium, with a seating capacity of 25,000, has room for a lot of fans (there will soon be an East stand expansion making overall capacity 30,000). Therefore tickets have to be sold! Also, technologically there ought to be a computerised database with fans' and supporters' details collected in order to maximise the organisation's knowledge of who attends matches. Hull FC would want to know what type of people do we have in our market? This knowledge would enable Hull FC to create offers specifically targeted in the right way to the right people….ie those most likely to buy tickets and attend matches/games to support their team.

Legal issues that would concern Hull FC include Acts such as the Town and Country Planning Act 1990 which would be responsible for planning permission (relevant to the forthcoming 5000 seat expansion at the KC stadium), and somebody such as John Prescott would have a casting 'vote' as to what developments actually go ahead. Also the Human Rights Article 14, 1998, relates to equal opportunities and non-discrimination issues, so players and staff members would be selected because of their ability to perform the job in hand and not rejected for reasons of prejudice. A further example to consider legally is that all players be subject to drug-testing; this would reduce the likelihood of players cheating by using performance enhancing drugs (NB Dwayne Chambers two year ban from athletics due to a positive drug test result). Should offenders be disciplined internally, or should the case go to Public Courts of Law? Ownership rights are legally binding and, at present, Hull City Council have these rights to Hull FC at the KC stadium. Finally, pricing (ie tickets or season passes) should be reasonable and affordable for all supporters.

In addition to these five 'PESTL' macro-environmental factors there are three more worth considering. Geographical is a question of territory. Hull FC is located on the north side of the river Humber, in Hull city, East Yorkshire, England, U.K. Within this same territory there are rivals and there are benefactors. Organisations compete for dominance, whilst at the same time looking at the bigger picture and benefiting other local enterprises by means of their own success. Demographically Hull has a working age population of 258,000. The East Riding of Yorkshire currently has 317,502 residents, of which 189,441 are of working age (ie 16-64 males, 16-59 females). All ages, genders, family sizes, incomes, occupations, educations and religions are to be considered however. The research could include questions sent out to all residents of Hull city, or even East Yorkshire to obtain details and opinions that could benefit Hull FC and its future prospects. Also there is the Psychographic element to consider. Here we look into personality, lifestyle, subculture and social class. Consumers are divided into groups on the basis of differences in their lifestyle ie how people live...what are their activities, interests and opinions?

The Micro-Environment - Competitors, Complementors, and Customers

There are both direct and indirect competitors. Hull Kingston Rovers are the direct competition to Hull FC. Based at 'Craven park', supporters for the Kingston Rovers support one team. Were there to be only one local team there would likely be twice the fan-base for that one team as rugby league supporters would have no option but to support the existing team. People change, people adapt, people evolve, consequently diversity arises where there might previously have been nothing. The indirect competition comes from non-local teams also in the Tetley's Rugby Super League, such as Bradford Bulls, Warrington Wolves, St Helens, Leeds and Wigan. Complementors are organisations whose presence and business operations benefit not only themselves, but also Hull FC. In the city of Hull there are many complementors of this sort eg 'The Deep' which offers discount prices for Hull FC season ticket holders. The Deep – a submarium - was designed by world-renowned architect Sir Terry Farrell and cost £45.5 million to build. There were over one million visitors in the first fifteen months of opening.

Also, 'Hull City' football team attract attention to the KC stadium – also home to Hull FC- thus gaining supporters' awareness. Concerts held at the KC stadium also attract awareness to a larger audience eg Sir Elton John performing there in the Summer of 2003. The 'Hull Stingrays' ice-hockey team make use of Hull Arena – home to an Olympic size Ice-skating arena – thus also increasing awareness of sport in the city of Hull. Another sporting asset to Hull are the 'Hull Vikings'-Speedway. Education-wise, Hull University is full of intelligent and educated students, lecturers and professors, thus enhancing the reputation of Hull as a city. This leads on to the next point….. 'City Image' is an organisation based in Hull whose goal is to enhance the status of Hull city and make Hull a top ten UK city permanently. This recently proved all the more challenging as Hull was nominated the worst town in the UK by an official 'Times' opinion poll! Another complementor is 'The Humber Bridge' aka 'The Gateway'. Completed in 1981 this is the third longest suspension bridge in the world, and has had over 100 million users. Hull is frequently symbolised by this piece of engineering, and provides a link to Lincolnshire on the other side of the River Humber for vehicles and pedestrians alike. Other assets to Hull are The Ferens Art Gallery, and the Museums Quarter valued at £5.1million and officially declared open by HRH The Duke of Gloucester in April 2003. The Waterfront boasts a yacht filled marina with over 300 berths, and is the location of festivals and events every year. Surrounding the marina area are bars, cafes, restaurants and shops.

Finally, Customers……There are four types of customer likely to be involved with Hull FC. There are locals and non-locals, and there are regulars and non-regulars. Between these four categories of customer, the research to be done could obtain specific details about which type of customer is going to provide the best business for Hull FC. The club slogan "100% Hull FC – Join the faithful" may be responsible for some customers attending matches – if they happen to believe in the slogan and what it stands for it could be a reason for their support.

Questions proposed for research – Who, what, why, where, when, how?

Who should we be targeting in order to discover what changes need to be made to maintain Hull FC's success? There are many people, clubs and sources that could provide valuable information…..Hull FC fans, players, coaches, management, and PR people for one. Also, local residents could have their say about how the changes have affected their lives (beneficially or otherwise). Other local sport's clubs could portray their opinions on Hull FC too eg Kingston Rovers (rugby league), The Tigers (football), The Stingrays (ice-hockey), and The Vikings (speedway).

What exactly is it that we want to find out? We wish to uncover people's attitudes, beliefs, ideas, and opinions about Hull FC; also we want to find out how to increase awareness of Hull FC by means of understanding the macro and micro-environments in which the organisation operates. What motivates people to be involved with Hull FC at all?

Why do we want to find this information out? In order to maintain the organisation's success we need to identify any barriers to usage and encourage users to remain involved with the club, and non-users to *become* involved and try out something that could be mutually beneficial to both organisation and user.

Where would this research take place? Initially, most would take place within the city of Hull itself as it is all related specifically to Hull FC and the KC stadium, Hull city, and related enterprises. Some would also take place beyond these bounds with regards to indirect competition ie other super-league rugby teams such as Leeds, Wigan or St Helens.

When would this research project go ahead? As soon as possible, by means of using data from the archives to create questions that would be appropriate and make progressive results to Hull FC today, this research would be responsible for influencing future prosperity so long as sufficient enough sources were to cooperate.

How would we: a) Increase awareness? By means of advertising in the local papers, radio, posters/flyers/programmes, and word-of-mouth, people would gain awareness.

b) Understand attitudes? By discovering the extent of loyalty that supporters and fans have to Hull FC. The slogan "100% Hull FC – join the faithful!" would indicate that those seriously involved with the club have a shared sense of loyalty.

c) Encourage usage? This would be a question of reaching out to every single person involved with the club and making everyone feel comfortable with their own level of involvement; evidently this would mean different things for each person.

d) Enhance motivational factors? Motivation comes in many forms and may include: results, territorial loyalty/pride, family/friends or other connections, provision of refreshments, price of tickets/season passes, personal aspirations eg to be a player, coach or manager, or even for the buzz of a new experience.

Proposed research methods

The questionnaire created must motivate the respondent to co-operate, become involved, and provide complete, honest and accurate answers. Timing is crucial to obtaining the desired results. Data collected ought to be both *Internal* (relevant to Hull FC eg data from sales invoices), and *External* (data from fans and the media. Sources which could be used include: commercial, governmental – census -, online databases, indexes, directories, or other syndicated services). By means of *Qualitative* data (exploration and description) we could use *Focus Groups* in Hull city with groups of no more than ten at any one time; or personal *Depth Interviews* using one technique from: projective, association, completion, construction, or expressive; or *Brainstorming* to get the creative responses flowing; or *Sampling*....Non-probability sampling comes in four types – convenience, judgemental, quota, or snowball.

Probability sampling also comes in four types – simple random, cluster, stratified, or systematic. One method would be chosen for the eventual questionnaire. The order of questions is most important as respondents need to feel at ease and not be bombarded with personal and sensitive issues that may cause unease. Questions should be specific, structured or unstructured, multiple-choice, or dichotomous. NB we as researchers would make the choice between a *Positivist* or *Interpretivist* approach. Also, by means of *Quantitative* data (experiment, exploration, and description) we could use statistical analysis, surveys, structured data collection, or interviews – either by mail, telephone, email, or personal at home or in the office. Street interviews are also an option, asking respondents who happen to be passing by at the time.

This last point leads on to '*Ethnography*' – the observation of customs, habits and differences between people in everyday situations. This very much applies to street interviewing. The 'Action Research Approach' involves five inter-connected activities, and they are: Action, Evaluation, Diagnosis, Analysis, and Feedback. They are all connected and the process can be linked to any one of these actions anytime in the process. *Ethics* is always an issue. The researcher must always respect respondents, and protect their anonymity. Respondents should not be misled or deceived, nor should they be embarrassed or harassed by the process of research.

In conclusion, Hull FC is the organisation and in order to maintain their success it is necessary to conduct research to analyse and make known how best to utilise the environment in which they operate; it is also necessary to take into account other organisations, competitive or altruistic, in or connected to Hull which are responsible for part of Hull FCs overall success.

Sources

Arnould, Price, Zinkhan (2004) *Consumers, International 2nd edition* –McGraw Hill
Hair, Bush, Ortinau (2003) *Marketing Research – within a changing information environment 2nd edition* – McGraw Hill Irwin
Malhotra N & Birks D (2003) *Marketing Research – An applied approach* – FT Prentice Hall
Monthly Digest of Statistics – No 697, January 2004
Oxford Bulletin of Economics and Statistics – Vol 66, February 2004, No1
www.hull.co.uk
www.hullcityafc.premiumtv.co.uk
www.hullfc.com
www.hullstingrays.co.uk
www.hullvikings.com
www.kcstadium.co.uk
www.nomisweb.co.uk
www.statistics.gov.uk
www.thedeep.co.uk
www.r11895.com/rugby-super-league.htm

Appendix 5 - Piracy and its effects on record sales in the Music Industry

Piracy is responsible for a dramatic decrease in record sales in the Music Industry today. Internet piracy, constituting of illegal file-sharing and downloading sites, is largely to blame. As a consequence of this, the Music Industry is losing its lifeblood through lost profits and fallen revenues as can be seen from some 2003 statistics – record sales in Britain fell by 6.1% from the previous years total, and in 2003 the US Music Industry lost $1.6bn due to internet piracy.[56] So the question arises "how can the Music Industry continue to support, financially, its budding artists?".

---

[56] The Financial Times (November 2003)

Research Purpose: This project proposal is for a *case study* to research the damaging effects (existing and potential) that internet piracy has on record sales today. Primary data will be collected, processed, analysed and compared to secondary data already existing with regards to piracy and the Music Industry. By doing this research specific problems could be targeted and specific people could be pin-pointed to determine how to a) decrease the amount of on-going piracy, b) prevent any further piracy from occurring, or c) reverse the effects, maintaining cash-flow in the Music Industry by enabling rightful record sales to be made. A common attitude that may be found amongst 'pirates' today would be: "Why should I pay for an album/single when it is available for free on the internet?" This is the problem. This is the purpose of the research – to discover how to reignite legitimate record sales, in the light of internet piracy.

Conceptual context: The media frequently portrays the Music Industry today, dominated by the 'Big five' – Sony, BMG, EMI, Warner, Universal - , as suffering the effects of piracy. International newspapers, such as The Financial Times, look at it from a business perspective and inform us how, statistically, record sales are down, profits are down, and piracy is on the increase. Other major (inter)national newspapers such as The Times, The Telegraph, The Guardian, and The Independent place these facts in the wider context…ie socially, for many, it is more than acceptable to be a part of the 'peer-to-peer' file-sharing community and acquire any type or amount of music of your taste at the touch of a button, irrespective of the fact that it is illegal. So it is a battle coming from the authorities trying to stamp out those who (technically) 'cheat' the system, although it can't be entirely 'cheating' as these sites are available to anybody who uses the internet. Local newspapers such as The Hull Daily Mail sometimes relates a bust to the public, such as December 2003 four people were arrested at Hull market and over £10,000 of illegal CDs, DVDs, and MP3s were seized by police.[57] Newspapers are full of facts, figures, statistics, and

---

[57] The Hull Daily Mail (10th December 2003)

information. So newspapers are a continuously updated source of intelligence whereby current information can be compared and contrasted with that of yesterday, last week, last month, or last year…..some may say "yesterday's news is no news!" the fact remains – the information remains useful regardless of its age.

In addition to newspapers, music-selling shops could be approached and stock counts of the current year and previous years too taken into consideration. Shops such as MVC, HMV, Virgin Megastores, Woolworths, WHSmiths sell records to the general public, therefore would be prime sources of inside information. An example of the difference between a bought album and a pirated album could be the following: "Twentysomething" by the artist "Jamie Cullum" costs £11.99 to buy from MVC. This same album could be obtained <u>free of charge</u> by downloading it from the internet, or by accessing a file-sharing site. Also, "The Clubber's Guide 2004" with tracks by various artists, bought from MVC costs £14.99 brand new. These tracks could be sought and obtained <u>free of charge</u> on-line!

Some examples of free internet sites a) for file-sharing, and b) for downloading, are as follows: a) <u>www.Kazaa.com</u>, <u>www.imesh.com</u>, <u>www.WinMX.com</u>; also <u>www.napster.com</u> is now legal as it has introduced a user fee; and b) <u>www.MP3.com</u>. Search engines could be used as well, eg by typing the words ' free downloads' or 'file sharing' into the word bar in any of the following: <u>www.google.co.uk</u>, <u>www.yahoo.co.uk</u>, <u>www.altavista.com</u>, <u>www.lycos.com</u>; the search engine would then produce the requested sites to visit. In doing so, the user would technically be walking a fine line between legal and illegal; this decision is entirely at the users discretion however.

Also, from the perspective of a market researcher, certain textbooks would be invaluable to refer to in order to obtain information about research methods, sampling techniques, statistical procedure/interpretation, ethics and more too. The textbooks that I have made use of for the purpose of this research proposal are as follows:

1)Zikmund, William G (2003) *Business Research Methods* – Thomson, SouthWestern 2) Birks D & Malhotra N (2002) *Marketing Research : An Applied Approach* –PrenticeHall,
3) Hair, Bush & Ortinau (2003)*Marketing Research Within a Changing Information Environment* – McGraw Hill,
4) Morris C (2000) *Quantitative Approaches in Business Studies* – FT Prentice Hall.

1) Zikmund provides a complete picture of the research procedure from conception of the project, through questionnaire design and data collection methods, to interpretation and analysis of gathered data. The book is clearly presented with clear learning objectives. 2) Birks and Malhotra puts the research into the broader perspective of the world we live in ie 'how will your research effect society/your objective?' Theory gathered from a questionnaire or survey is turned into hard facts, and this book enables the researcher to undertake this process. 3) Hair, Bush and Ortinau also puts the theory gathered from research into a wider picture ' how does it relate to the world we live in?' The book enables the user to interpret/translate the collected data into practical terms ie how to organise focus groups and in-depth interviews and then put the information in perspective with related issues. 4) Morris provides some fundamental learning objectives with regards to theory, data collection and quantitative data approaches. This book provides the foundation for more detailed research approaches as the researcher becomes progressively more advanced.

Some ethical points to take into consideration throughout the course of the case study would include the '7 C's' that ought to occur between market researcher and client. They are: communication, cooperation, confidence, candour, closeness, continuity, and creativity.[58] When put into action these '7 C's'

---

[58] Malhotra & Birks (2003:51) Marketing Research – an applied approach

> Depth interviews – £7,500;
> Focus Groups – £8,000;
> Telephone Interviews – £2,500;
> Street interviews - £1,500;

Total: £22,000

The expense would be repaid in due course as the music industry regains composure and record sales rise once again like a phoenix from the flames.

Ethics: Certain ethical issues need to be taken into consideration whilst conducting research in order to achieve fair and unbiased results. The following are some of the considerations to take into account: Subjects reserve the right to expect something in return from the research; Individuals must give their full consent to taking part in the research and being interviewed; The researcher must respect the respondents' confidentiality/privacy and measures ought to be taken to ensure the data gathered is not misused in any way; Data collected should be safeguarded; The manner in which the research is reported is important and must conform to acceptable standards eg those set by ESOMAR; The European Society for Opinion and Marketing Research (ESOMAR) produce a code of conduct in order to protect the interests of all research stakeholders; In general, for each of the stages of marketing research design process the same four stakeholders – client, researcher, respondent, and public – should act honourably and respect their responsibilities to one another;[60] The act of disguising the true nature of the survey by either 'sugging' – the deliberate act of disguising a sales pitch, or 'frugging' – the deliberate act of disguising a fundraising attempt, would be a serious breach of conduct.

Most market research would generally be conducted by commercial firms ie those for-profit only, divided between the two categories of : industrial research organisations (external suppliers), and departments within organisations (internal

---

[60] Malhotra & Birks (2003:680)

5) General public – could be any of the above four (random sample).

The groups would be selected by Non-probability Judgemental sampling. Each group would take one hour to take place. Therefore, timescale for focus groups = two days – three one day, two the next. Costing = £8,000. Ethical issues to consider for focus groups include 'drugging'...should the researcher provide alcoholic drinks to help subjects relax and contribute more openly to the session? Or would this be unethical? Also, there should not be any usage of audio or video recorders, or two-way mirrors, in the focus group without the consent of all respondents.

There could also be a Non-probability Convenience sample taken in the form of telephone interviews....selecting from a phone book as feels convenient. Maybe 250-500 calls, lasting 5-10 minutes each asking relevant questions to the receiver. These could be completed within three weeks. Costing for maximum of 500 calls would total at approximately £2,500. It would also be possible to conduct street interviews (750 – 1,000) and take some surveys to the street and ask every n'th member of the public to please spare a moment of their time and help the research. If each survey takes 10 minutes to complete then, at a maximum, they could be completed over the period of four weeks (ie five hours/day). Costing would be approximately £1,500. Street interviewing is also known as 'guerilla ethnography'.[59]

Timescale: Questionnaires – two weeks;
Depth interviews – three weeks;
Focus Groups – two days;
Telephone interviews – three weeks;
Street interviews – four weeks;
Total: *Fourteen weeks*

Costing: Questionnaires – £2,500;

---

[59] Malhotra & Birks (2003:151) Marketing Research....

A sampling frame of between 2,500-5,000 sources would be used, the majority being in the form of individuals filling out and returning questionnaires, either being sent out with a returnable Freepost envelope or being handed out personally on a one-to-one visit/session. Eg 3,000 questionnaires sent out initially to the following two broad categories of people: A) existing and known file-sharing/downloading users. B) potential (those unknown to) file-share/download users ie 'legitimate' music fans. More specifically the strategically significant target group would include: the general public, Managers and staff of various record shops such as MVC, HMV, Virgin Megastores, etc.., personnel in the Music Industry such as producers, artists, and agents…those 'in the know'. So questionnaires would be sent out, selected by Systematic probability sampling, to the general music-appreciating public and to Music Industry personnel. From 3,000 questionnaires I would expect a return of at least 750 completed questionnaires. Each questionnaire would be designed to take no longer than 15minutes to complete, and a completion and return time of two weeks would be taken into account before following up and collecting data. Costing of 3,000 questionnaires would be approximately £2,500.

Also, In-depth Interviews would be conducted – between 100-300 each lasting 20 minutes, so a maximum timescale for interviews of 100 hours taking place over a course of one month. Interviewees would be of the same types as for questionnaire method. Costing would be more expensive….approximately £7,500. Another method of data-collection is Focus Groups. I propose to conduct 5 focus groups, each of 10 people, directed at the following five categories:

1) Existing, known file-sharer/downloader & Music Industry personnel.
2) Existing, known file-sharer/downloader & non-Music Industry personnel.
3) Potential (unknown to) file-share/download user & Music Industry personnel.
4) Potential (unknown to) file-share/download user & non-Music Industry personnel.

24) Are you happy to continue buying merchandise in the knowledge that many people are getting the same merchandise for free?

"Thankyou for your time – your responses are of great value to us!" (to be included at the end of the questionnaire).

Most of the above 24 questions simply require a 'yes' or 'no' answer, however there are some which would require an opinion and need to be elaborated on, therefore could provide a basis to be included in the focus groups and in-depth interviews where participants would be able to express more elaborate responses, opinions and attitudes and get involved with a more discursive approach than that created by a questionnaire/survey.

Research Methods: This project will be a case study, the case being 'the damaging effects of piracy on record sales in the Music Industry today'. Throughout the course of this project both Qualitative and Quantitative data will be collected and analysed. The former to express thoughts, ideas, attitudes and opinions; the latter to express statistics, and hard data in the form of: numbers of file-sharing/downloading users, numbers of records sold, and cost of singles/albums/records – a) to the customer, b) to the Music Industry. From an ethical perspective, Quantitative data would produce a more definite set of results because there are established and consistent procedures of analysis for this type. Conversely, for Qualitative data there are no consistent and established procedures of analysis, consequently data collected is more open to interpretation. It would be important to minimise sampling and non-sampling error by being as concise as possible throughout the research procedure. An Interval scale of measurement will be used, thus enabling the researcher to compare the price differences from one point in time to another point in time. eg 2003 profits could be directly contrasted to 1998 profits in the Music Industry. Also a Nominal scale of measurement could be used to differentiate between 1-those who file-share/download on the internet, and 2-those who do NOT file-share/download on the internet.

suppliers). Each researcher has the potential to misuse or abuse their marketing research by, for example, misrepresenting the research findings. The following four ethical dilemmas would also apply to market research (1) There is no need to collect primary data when secondary data alone would address the problem (and vice versa). (2) There is no need to use secondary data that are not applicable. (3) Secondary data should not be used that has been gathered through morally questionable means. (4) The researcher should not compromise the anonymity of customer details on databases.

Summary: This is a project proposal for a case study researching how the number of record sales in today's Music Industry has been damaged by piracy and the free internet downloading and file-sharing revolution. The purpose of the project is to compile data that would establish specifically where the fall in sales stems from, thereby taking action and reversing this trend and maintaining profits in the record industry. Research methods to be put into action for this project include questionnaires, surveys, in-depth interviews (personal and telephone), focus groups, and street interviews. The proposed target respondents would include those who: file-share or download music products online; and those who do not file-share or download music products online; music industry personnel; non-music industry personnel; and the general public. Total estimated timescale = 14 weeks; Total estimated costing = £22,000.

Bibliography

Birks D & Malhotra N (2002) *Marketing Research : An Applied Approach* –PrenticeHall,
Hair, Bush & Ortinau (2003)*Marketing Research Within a Changing Information Environment* – McGraw Hill,
Morris C (2000) *Quantitative Approaches in Business Studies* – FT Prentice Hall.
Saunders, Lewis, & Thornhill (1997) *Research Methods for Business Students* - Pitman Publishing
The Financial Times (December 2003 – January 2004)
The Guardian (November 2003)
Hull Daily Mail (December 2003)
Zikmund, William G (2003) *Business Research Methods* – Thomson, SouthWestern
www.imesh.com
www.kazaa.com
www.mp3.com
www.napster.com
www.WinMx.com

Appendix 6 - Compare and contrast the approach of any three paradigms to the role of management theory and practice. Chosen paradigms are: Interpretivism, Functionalism, and Critical Theory.

Interpretivism is a paradigm which focuses mainly on culture (internal to an organisation), and correspondingly the term 'clan' is recognised and utilised as a regular metaphor for this paradigm. Areas of development, progress and focus include group dynamics, understanding and management of identity. There are numerous theories specifically relevant to interpretivism and they include: Human Relations (Mayo), Organisational Culture (Yanow), and Excellence Literature (Peters). These will be looked into in greater depth at a later stage of this essay. The paradigm also involves: Anthropology, Social Psychology, Psychoanalysis, and Micro-Sociology (Geertz, Yanow, and Peters have influence in this area). With regards to shaping patterns of identity, managers of this paradigm-type are leaders or anthropologists.[61]

Functionalism focuses on (internal) decision-making; the metaphor here used is bureaucracy; the main emphasis is on control, efficiency, and problem solving. Related theories are Taylorism and classical administrative management (Fayol), Resource based view (Grant/Barney), Stakeholder theories (Freeman), Cognitive and systems approaches (Simon/Senge). With regards to shaping patterns of attention, problem setting and solving the manager is seen as ruler (boss). Ontological and Epistemological viewpoints within the managerialist matrix involve functionalism as : realism/ instrumentalism, positivism, determinism and nomothetic.[62]

Critical Theory focuses on culture and (social) citizenship. The manager here is seen as social democrat. The Frankfurt School – originators of critical theory - consisting of Adorno, Horkheimer,

---

[61] Andresani G (2004) Lecture 6 notes, blackboard
[62] Andresani G (2004) Lecture 6 notes, blackboard

et al. were forced to leave their native Germany because of the Nazis. The second generation of the Frankfurt school formed throughout the 1950s/60s eg Marcuse, Habermas. Scholars and practitioners should aim at achieving emancipation in theory and practice. There is focus on cultural analysis and targets of critique : 'Scientism' (positivism/ fuctionalism) and 'technocratic' power. An example of a theory by Habermas is on liberation (ie emancipatory cognitive interest) from unecessary suffering. He advocates that Social problems should be solved by open discussion and argumentation. A well developed 'public sphere' is the necessary condition for social democratic settlement.

Habermas contributed that in organisational settings, conditions should be put in place for 'unconstrained' (rational) discussion. Individuals and groups (clans) should steer systems (organisations and institutions) by putting in place (social) democratic procedures eg German codetermination , not the other way round. There is a notion of social citizenship/ democracy. He places an emphasis (Kantian) on ethics: freedom from power (bureaucracy) and economic systems. Strengths of the critical theory paradigm include: effort to reconcile (interpretive and neo-institutionalism) with technical (functionalism and free market) interests by focusing on (emancipation from) power. Goal is establishing (social) justice and democracy in the workplace. Weaknesses of the paradigm include: 'Ideal speech' situation seen as utopian/ difficult to achieve. European (social) democracy criticised by poor (third and fourth) worlds for at least helping the US domination or not doing enough to (socially) democratise its institutions. Pervasiveness of power and social structures as well as benefits of bureaucracy are neglected.[63]

Having looked at the three paradigms in a nutshell, it is necessary to place them into practical context. By using a case study 'The coffee clash' and bureaucracy too, these three paradigms will be analysed and put into context.

---

[63] Andresani G (2004) Lecture 6 notes, blackboard

Case study

'The coffee clash' involves Starbucks and its choice to trade in fair trade coffee. So, decision-making, the focus of functionalism, is the first to be put into practice......the decision to trade in fair trade coffee from farmer to consumer. As for interpretivism and critical theory the focus is on culture. Coffee is an established part of our culture, and everywhere in the world too. The culture of waking up first thing in the morning and drinking fresh roast coffee. The case study focuses on numerous issues within the coffee trade and some are as follows: quality control, fair trade, other innovation, sweatshop labour, charitable causes, leadership, alternatives eg Colombian drug trading, organic and environmentally friendly produce. If we analyse these issues in terms of the three chosen paradigms we find common threads to the case. In terms of quality control this is a process of decision-making (functionalism); fair trade is sociological, so it benefits the whole clan (interpretivism); innovation is a case for individuals taking the lead (manager as leader = interpretivism); sweatshop labour is a cultural issue and involves manager as boss, in a system of pure bureaucracy (so functionalism); charitable causes involve social democracy so here we are talking about critical theory; leadership relates to the interpretive paradigm; alternative trade is all about trial and error, some times an absolute ruler would preside over the proceedings (functionalism), other times a more socially democratic procedure would be the norm (critical theory); finally organic/environmentally friendly produce...this is clearly sociological and would involve manager as anthropologist or social democrat, so interpretivism and critical theory apply to this practice. So we can see here that the coffee case study is linked to all three paradigms in some way.[64]

Also, it is necessary to examine the concept of bureaucracy as there is some division between the paradigms concerning this concept. Functionalism has a strong leaning towards

---

[64] Roosevelt M & Huatusco (2004) The coffee clash – Time Inside Business

bureaucracy and manager as ruler, or manager as boss. The focus here of decision-making would be very much top-down ie management make the decisions, and employees merely implement them, having been given instructions as to what to do. Compared with interpretivism and critical theory whose focuses are chiefly concerned with culture, manager in critical theory is very much social democrat, and manager in interpretivism is very much leader and anthropologist, the three paradigms can be seen to differ vastly in terms of bureaucracy. The managerialist paradigm looks to maintain the status quo, therefore a degree of functionalist bureaucracy would apply; and the critical paradigm looks to change the status quo, therefore critical theory and the Starbuck's coffee case would apply, as management are on the continuous lookout to change things for the better.

Also, in practice Critical theory could apply to Socialist Feminist Theory. Gender is a constitutive element of social relationships based on perceived differences by the sexes. Gender is a make-up of behavioural and cultural constructs ie male and female, as opposed to sex which is of biological construct (chromosomes and anatomy). Gender is a primary way of signifying relationships of power; there are different forms of men's interest in the domination of women; also, there is the issue of exploitation under patriarchy and under capitalism; the 'glass ceiling' is related to women's struggles ie attitudes, customs, legal constraints block women's entrance and/or success in the world of work. Remedies include reform, education, and the removal of discrimination. This comes within critical theory.[65]

Evolution, ethology, and anthropology all contribute to our understanding of feminist theory. The role of the male is to impregnate the female who necessarily undergoes the process of childbirth. Different cultures treat this process in very different ways eg Mbuti pygmees are casual with regard to childbirth; Alor people in Indonesia treat the event as everyday; Aborigines of Tasmania continue to work hard every day even when heavily pregnant; the Amazons contained many females in its armies;

---

[65] Afanassieva M (2004) Lecture notes – Feminist Theory

Burundi people are suited to hard labour, women too ; British females would once have a large role to play in agricultural work. It is said that it is men that want children and women who bear and rear children. Family and marriage are important institutions for us.[66]

So, a recap of the paradigms in their broader theoretical picture before looking at them in greater depth:

Ontology and Epistemology are two branches of philosophy covering a wide area of academic theory and their meanings can be related to managerial practice in Organisations. The selected paradigms contain certain philosophies too, and they are: *Interpretivism* – Nominalism, Anti-positivism, Voluntarism, and Ideographic; *Functionalism* – Realism, Instrumentalism, Positivism, Determinism/ Nomothetic; *Critical theory* – Nominalism, Anti-positivism, Voluntarism, Determinism and Ideographic. Thus their fundamental similarities can be seen.[67]

So, the three paradigms in greater depth…..

Interpretivism

In the early 1800s the term Social positivism was coined with regards to the theory that if universal laws can be discovered for the physical and natural world they can also be found for the social or human world. The term evolved through the mid 1800s as Evolutionary positivism, to the late 1800s as Critical positivism/empiriocriticism. The philosopher Kant said that 'knowing depends on a priori knowledge' , therefore the interpretive paradigm could also be recognised as neo-Kantian/neo-Idealist. Another philosopher Simmel progressed the argument in favour of content and form studying both meaning (values, beliefs, feelings of lived experiences) and the artefacts that embody meaning. Kant coined the word 'verstehen' which Weber translated to 'bergreifen' meaning that

---

[66] Oakley A (1974) Myths of woman's place
[67] Andresani G (2004) Lecture 7 notes, blackboard

they were against the notion that the sense-based facts of nature, seen by positivists as external to human actors, could simply be grasped. What we know of this world arises through interpreting our sense perceptions, not from an uninterrupted grasping of them.[68]

Concluding remarks on the interpretive paradigm : 'interpretive work is supported on its own merits, rather than merely in relation to positivist thought. As a consequence, interpretive research methods for accessing and analyzing data (eg observing, interviewing, content-analysis, semiotics, ethnomethodology, metaphor analysis) are themselves becoming better understood and judged according to their own presuppositions, rather than against positivist scientific criteria for validity and reliability which they cannot meet.[69]

Disagreements and controversies arise within Interpretivism over the following dichotomies: objectivity/subjectivity, etic (outsider) and emic (insider) research, generalizable and context-specific research, focus and breadth, and level of depth.

Examples of these dichotomies are as follows…..*objectivity* – a set of sounds in a language may be heard differently by speakers of different languages. Also the taste of foods is *subjective* eg dog meat is not eaten in the United States, but there they eat beef, Indians revere the cow and consequently do not eat beef, and in some African countries dog meat is considered a delicacy. Moving on to the *etic/emic* dichotomies, with the former, cultural research includes any study qualitative or quantitative where the conceptual categories are imposed by the researcher, rather than initiated by the cultural member who is being studied. Malinowski stated that with emic the idea was "to seek to grasp the native's point of view, his relation to life, to realize his vision of the world". Geertz said "an anthropologist's task is that of a

---

[68] Hatch M J/Yanow D (2003) Organization theory as an interpretive science
[69] Hatch M J/Yanow D (2003) Org……..

translator", and with regard to 'emic': " the trick is to figure out what the devil they think they are up to".[70]

Generalizable and context specific knowledge; Geertz said "the task of an anthropologist is to produce an interpretation of the way a people lives". NB ethnographies cover this subject area. He also stated that cultural homogeneity cannot be assumed, therefore it is a fallacy to generalize about a whole culture.

The Interpretative paradigm gives us a worldview and an overall general perspective on the way organisations operate.[71]

Functionalism

Positivism is tied in with functionalism. The liberal revolution in Eastern Europe had profound effects worldwide eg 1989 the Berlin wall was torn down, and also in 1989 the Tiananman square massacre occurred in Beijing. The third way was thus formulated, incorporating radical structuralism, subjectivism, and humanism. Talcott Parsons predicted in 1964 a theory of evolutionary universals which at the time was criticized but since the time has been an accurate prediction of real events. Scott concluded that there are two different discourses that form the backbone of Organizational Theory - Sociological and Managerial.[72]

The spirit of the progressive era was congruent with the promise of systems to promote 'progress of equality'. A functionalist outlook is quoted here: "there is not a man, machine or operation or system in this shop that stands entirely alone. Each one, to be valued rightly, must be viewed as part of a whole". (American Machinist 03/03/1904). Also "you must have a cost system. You can't retain the respect of the manufacturing public if you don't

---

[70] Martin J (2003) Meta-theoretical controversies in studying organizational culture
[71] Martin J (2003) Meta……
[72] Shenhav Y (2003) The historical and epistemological foundations of organization theory

have one.....a cost system is as necessary to your industrial prestige as a pair of pants to your personal dignity" (American Machinist 03/07/1913).

Weber examined different aspects of rationality eg action, decision, and systematized world views; and applied rationalization – the cultivation of rationality in western society in particular – to diverse spheres of life such as religion, law, economics, and music (Weber 1921/1968). Weber also decided that with regard to contradictions for sociology 'most noticeable are those between the universality of heuristic devices, on the one hand, and the idiosyncrasy of social processes on the other; between the intentionality of action, on the one hand, and its unintended consequences on the other; between Kantian-like 'objectives' ideal types and the subjective meaning of action.[73]

Critical theory

All paradigms strongly attack instrumental rationality and reject (neoclassical/ shareholding) Economic logic ie managers are effectively servants of wealthy owners NB Friedman "the only obligation of managers is to their shareholders". Progressive Politics involves: power, conflict, ethics and democracy, instead of efficiency, profitability, flexibility and control.[74]

Burrell and Morgan decided on the critical notion that: "the individual creates the world in which he lives". Habermas's theory contains three important concerns in organisational studies. 1) the aspiration of management knowledge to be scientific. 2) the fragmentation of methodologies within organisational studies. 3) the scope for recognizing and combining the distinctive contributions of different forms of knowledge. NB New Organisational Forms (NOF's) illustrate Habermas's theory.

---

[73] Shenhav Y (2003) The historical......
[74] Andresani G (2004) Lecture 7 notes, blackboard

Postmodernism is at the heart of this critique and is the objection that taken for granted, modernist truths of 'objective knowledge', 'rigorous analysis', 'independent scrutiny' et al. aspire to be totalizing. Postmodernism unsettles these 'truths'. The Critical Modernist Alternative "Critical modernists", Habermas included, "share a postmodern scepticism about value-free knowledge, yet seek to retain and revive the spirit of the Enlightenment in the face of what are regarded as the perversions of reason, including the power invested in scientific authority by systemic modernism."[75]

Habermas points to the experience of (uneccessary) frustration and suffering which , he contends, stimulates yet also frustrates a desire to 'throw off relations' that 'repress without necesssity'. Critical science strives to expose the unreasoned, political basis of this givenness in contrast to 'empirical-analytical' and 'historical-hermeneutic' sciences. Habermas argues "all validity claims become imminent to particular discourses. They are simultaneously absorbed into the totality of some one of the blindly occurring discourses and left at the mercy of the 'hazardous play' amongst these discourses as each over-powers the other".[76]

In conclusion, the three paradigms Interpretivism, Functionalism, and Critical Theory, have their similarities and have their differences. Fundamental philosophical similarities include: Nominalism, Voluntarism, and Determinism. Differences between the three in terms of management are: manager as leader/anthropologist (interpretivism), manager as ruler/boss (functionalism), and manager as social democrat (critical theory). When put in perspective of the live case study ' Starbuck's coffee trade', their relevance becomes apparent and the situation can be analysed throughout its intricacies of dealings. Finally, the question 'Cui bono?' (whose interest?) should be answered….. Interpretivism equates to managers and (organisational) stakeholders/community; Functionalism equates

---

[75] Willmott H (2003) Organization theory as a critical science?
[76] Willmott H (2003) Org………

to Top managers; and Critical Theory equates to social citizenship.[77]

---

[77] Andresani G (2004) Lecture 9 notes - blackboard

Bibliography

Afanassieva M (2004) *Lecture notes* - blackboard

Alvesson M & Willmott H (2003) *Studying Management Critically* – SAGE London

Andresani G (2004) *Lecture notes* – blackboard

Clegg S (2002) *Central currents in organization studies* – Vols 1,2,3 – SAGE London

Hassard J & Parker M eds (1994) *Towards a new theory of organizations* – Routledge London / New York

Morgan G (1997) *Images of organizations* – SAGE -Thousand Oaks – London

Oakley A (1974) *Myths of woman's place* – Penguin books London

Reed M I (1992) *The sociology of organizations: themes, perspectives and prospects* Harvester Wheatsheaf – New York

Tsoukas H & Knudsen C eds (2003) *The Oxford handbook of organization theory* – Oxford University Press – Oxford / New York

Appendix 7 – Logistics Management

Q1) The best definition would be an entirely subjective opinion and decision to make. In the light of which I prefer the Council of Logistics Management definition 'That part of the supply chain process that plans, implements, and controls the efficient, effective flow and storage of goods, services, and related information from point of origin to point of consumption in order to meet customer requirements'[78].

To me this definition represents something specific within the overall configuration of the field of Logistics Management ie 'that part of the supply chain process'. The functions are also detailed within this definition 'that plans, implements, and controls' and also the quality is detailed 'efficient, effective flow and storage'. Specifically related to 'goods, services and related information', then the path or direction of all the above is also detailed 'from point of origin to point of consumption' ie the entire course that will be taken from inception to consumption, and finally the goal is stated ' to meet customer requirements'.

So, all in all a comprehensive definition accounting for the many different assets, requirements, obligations, directions, and operations of Logistics Management.

My understanding of Logistics Management comes largely from driving on motorways/highways and observing countless numbers of corporate lorries driving along with the words 'Logistics of so-and-so company....keeping your business in shape', or something along these lines. Therefore it could be said that this module will be the first 'insider insight' that I learn about logistics management.

Q2) Of significant import to a business is the ethical stance and values instilled throughout the organisation. Canadian Tire shares the following:

---

[78] Coyle, Bardi, Langley (2003:39) The Management of Business Logistics

Across the enterprise, we share a compelling vision: We are a growing, innovative network of interrelated businesses, achieving extraordinary results through extraordinary people. We touch the lives of more people in more ways every day.

Canadian Tire's vision comes to life through our Team Values:

We are *learners*... who thrive in a challenging and fast-paced environment.

We are *committed* ... to operate with honesty, integrity and respect.

We are *owners* ... with a passion to continuously improve.

We are *driven* ... to help customers achieve their goals.

We are *accountable* ... to ourselves and each other.

We are *leaders* ... who perform with heart[79].

The Canadian Tire Way is our foundation and inspiration that will continue to guide our future growth and success

Wal-Mart also practices ethics and values:

Sam Walton's 3 Basic Beliefs the company was built on.

Sam Walton built Wal-Mart on the revolutionary philosophies of excellence in the workplace, customer service and always having the lowest prices. We have always stayed true to the Three Basic Beliefs Mr. Sam established in 1962:

1. Respect for the Individual

---

[79] http://www2.canadiantire.ca/CTenglish/vision.html

2. Service to Our Customers
3. Strive for Excellence

Respect the individual 'Our people make the difference' is not a meaningless slogan - it's a reality at Wal-Mart. We are a group of dedicated, hardworking, ordinary people who have teamed together to accomplish extraordinary things. We have very different backgrounds, different colors and different beliefs, but we do believe that every individual deserves to be treated with respect and dignity."

Service to our customers we want our customers to trust in our pricing philosophy and to always be able to find the lowest prices with the best possible service. We're nothing without our customers.

Strive for Excellence New ideas and goals make us reach further than ever before. We try to find new and innovative ways to push our boundaries and constantly improve[80].

Wal-Mart is of American and International divergence, whereas Canadian Tire is based throughout Canada only. In the light of which Wal-Mart could be said to generate a broader revenue and clientele than Canadian Tire. However, an advantage to Canadian Tire is that they offer on-line shopping facilities to consumers therefore making the selection and purchase experience a whole world more convenient as people are able to shop from home if so desired.

Q3) York, North Yorkshire, England (UK). My home town holds host to a vast diversity of assets economical, social, political, artistical, technological, educational, and many others too. For example a major economical advantage within York is the rail transport industry. Over 600 million passengers pass

---

[80] http:www.walmartstores.com/wmstore/wmstores/Mainabout.jsp?BV.....

through York every year by train. The main two company-based HQ's situated in York are Great North Eastern Railways, and Arriva Trains Northern. The latter of which currently thrives on a £308 million turnover and runs 1275 miles of track, transporting 100 000 passengers per day and employing 2300 regional staff to manage the system[81].

Education features strongly in York with the university rating as the highest outside of Oxbridge and London, ie within the top 5 in the country. York city football team attracts greater crowds than results, but many loyal fans remain true to their home team.

Food and drink industry in York sees major organisations such as Nestle with a recent £150 million investment, Trebor Bassett (part of Cadbury Schweppes) employs 500 staff, and major breweries include Tadcaster's John Smiths, also Scottish Courage, Samuel Smiths, and Coors. Also Theakston's, Black Sheep Brewery and the Cropton Brewery are all major North Yorkshire assets.

Two logistical advantages to York city would be the major supply routes by road and rail as illustrated by the previous rail information, thus enabling products and consumers to travel between places eg factory to vendor/retailer, or home to work. Secondly the quantity of quality businesses in and around the York area amount to a marked benefit for the region.

Two logistical disadvantages for the area would include the River Ouse running through the middle of the city thus giving an expectation of using the waterway for commercial shipping advantages. In fact the river is no longer used as a major commercial shipping facility, therefore this could be a disadvantage. Secondly for sports fans the city's football team is never too successful, therefore this aspect could reduce some people's logistical perception of the region.

---

[81] http://www.york-england.com/economy.shtml

Q4) From a marketing perspective what product characteristics affect logistics costs? Using the examples as requested of Sleeman's, Molson's and Labatt's it is possible to see how specific prices vary depending on logistical reasons such as product format eg bottled, canned, kegged or on tap; also dependent on factors such as labelling type, packaging and marketing image. Logistical costs include the following specific examples taken from source:

Sleemans clear 6 can – Sleeman brewery CAD$10.99

Sleeman clear 6 bottle – Sleeman brewery CAD$9.99

Sleeman cream ale 5 litre keg CAD$20.99

Sleeman cream ale 6 can CAD$11.29

Sleeman cream ale 6 bottle CAD$10.29

Sleeman cream ale 12 bottle CAD$18.99

Sleeman honey brown lager 6 bottle CAD$10.29

Sleeman honey brown lager 12 bottle CAD$18.99

Sleeman original dark 6 bottle CAD$10.29

Sleeman selection pack 12 bottle CAD$19.49

We can see from this that the price of canned Sleemans is consistently higher than bottled Sleemans. Logistically this could be due to production costs and graphics used for the labelling/packaging.

Molson Canadian 6 can CAD$9.49

Molson Canadian 12 can CAD$17.99

The Green Dragon

Molson Canadian 16 can CAD$19.99

Molson Canadian 24 can CAD$34.99

Molson Canadian 8 can CAD$13.29

Molson Canadian 5 litre keg CAD$19.99

Molson Canadian Light 12 can CAD$16.99

Molson Canadian Light 6 can CAD$9.99

We can see from this that Molson produce canned and not bottled produce. The value works out cheaper the more items per purchase ie 24 cans is CAD$0.99 cheaper than 2 x 12 cans.

Labatt Blue 6 cans CAD$9.49

Labatt Blue 12 cans CAD$17.99

Labatt Blue 24 cans CAD$34.99

Labatt Blue 8 cans CAD$13.29

Labatt Blue Light 12 can CAD$17.99

Labatt Blue Light 24 can CAD$34.99

Labatt Blue Light 8 can CAD$13.29

Labatt Lite 12 can CAD$17.99

Labatt maximum ice 12 can CAD$18.49

Labatt sterling 6 can CAD$10.29

Labatt Wildcat 12 can CAD$15.29

Labatt Wildcat 8 can CAD$10.79[82]

Likewise with Labatt, produce is sold by the can not by the bottle. Costs are slightly favourable with a larger amount ordered in the long run.

Q5) Perform an analysis of two brands of bottled water looking for evidence that supply chains and the marketing mix are closely linked. Dasani and Aquafina provide two examples. Product: bottled water for both. Price: $1.75/bottle (350ml). Promotion: advertisement by means of supermarket promotions, tv adverts, posters, billboards, buses and more. Place: produced and manufactured specifically in factories and distributed to retail outlets, vendors, marketing campaigns and consumers.

The marketing mix consists of these four aspects in particular and supply chains involve the process of supplying in order to meet up with demand.

The challenges in terms of inbound logistics for these two brands would separate the one from the other...Dasani has been involved in a major scandal over the last two or three years....the water at source had been found to come from a tap-water source as opposed to a natural spring. Therefore coca-cola were sued and forced to withdraw all Dasani from the UK market. This event tarnished their reputation and meant a significant loss of sales for the company. Outbound logistics problems involve the distribution of the brands (more difficult for Dasani in light of the scandal). Aquafina has more of a fun image.....Squakafina as it could be called. This brand has been established on the Canadian market for many years and people have come to trust the product over this period of time. Considerations for Aquafina? They sell the product in many different sizes and quantities, the water is pure, the price is right,

---

[82] www.nsliquor.ns.ca

and people trust the product. Therefore all in all a quality product with logistics being exercised in all fairness.

Appendix 8 - *Evaluate the net economic benefits that two specific mainland European regions have received, during this decade, from UK and Eire based low-cost airlines establishing continental European-based operational bases. These regions will be in European countries such as France and Belgium, where EasyJet and Ryanair <u>respectively have established routes to and from the UK and Eire.</u>*

"Without doubt the tragic events of September 11 have had an unprecedented, devastating and immediate impact on all segments of our industry (airports, airlines, handling agents, flight caterers, and air navigation service providers) with unpredictable economic and social consequences. The aviation industry is currently beset with the immense challenges of coordinating and funding new security measures and finding a solution to the war/terrorism insurance crisis."[83] (Philippe G E Hannon – Director General ACI Europe)

With this in mind we will evaluate the Spanish regions Andalucia, Catalunia and the regions Basel and Zurich in Switzerland. The geopolitics between the two will be scrutinised. Specifically, the city of Granada with Ryanair flight routes direct from London (Stansted), and the city of Barcelona with Easyjet flight routes direct from London (Gatwick). Likewise, the new-established Euroairport at Basel-Mulhouse contains direct flights to and from London (Stansted and Luton). Zurich being locally accessible to Basel is also a major consideration.

---

[83] http://www.aci-europe.org/upload/144181672002aci%20july%202002%20all%20policy.pdf#search='easyjet%20ceo'

What else could there be in Espana to effect all airways and national infrastructure? 911, it seems, was not enough; March 11th 2004 saw the Madrid train bombings, killing 192 commuters in the early morning rush hour and injuring over 1500 others. Effects still being felt from this tragedy are today linked to al Qaeda, and the repercussions saw an immediate change in national outlook. In came the instantaneous election of Jose Luis Rodriguez Zapatero Head of Government, President and Prime Minister as of 17 April 2004, leader of the Spanish Socialist Workers party. Mr Zapatero instantly sought negotiations with the violent Basque Separatist group Eta in order to enhance national peace, also withdrawing all Spanish troops from Iraq. Optimistic about Spain's future, seeing 400 000 new jobs created last year, and the economy rise 3%, his policies are a mixture both of caution and complacency[84].

So how does this background relate to the question at hand?

Catalonia is Spain's economic powerhouse. The inclusive regions Barcelona, Biscay, Madrid, Navarre, and Oviedo produce *over half* the country's industrial output. The Spanish economy is Europe's fifth largest today accounting for 9% EU output. Andalucian tourism alone accounts for 4% GDP and 10% Spain's workforce are currently employed here. Early 90's Spain saw massive recession in the EU. Output and investment decreased, public deficit went up, bankruptcies and inflation rocketed. Between the years 1995-1999 Spain received $22.8bn from the EU to improve specifically, the infrastructure, roads, airports, waterways and communications. Notably, 30% Spanish industries are foreign-owned, 50% food production in Spain is French owned. The largest companies are state owned and loss-making. Spain's most important industries are tourism, chemicals, petrochemicals, heavy industry, food and beverages, metals and manufacturing, textiles and apparel, automobiles, medical equipment, clay and refractory products. Major agricultural products include grain, vegetables, olives, wine

---

[84] Financial Times (Tuesday June 14th 2005:p6) Special Report 'Spain'

grapes, sugar beets, citrus, beef, pork, poultry, fish and dairy products[85]. Spain's wine exports by 2004 figured at €1.55bn compared to Australia's €1.57bn. Competition from New World Wines is spurring Spanish winemakers to improve both quality of product and positioning of their brands.

Spanish factfile 2005[86]

Area: 504, 782 sq km – Population: 40,341 462 - Population growth rate: 0.15%
Birth rate: 10.1 births/1,000 population - Death rate: 9.63 deaths/1,000 population
Net migration rate: 0.99 migrants/1,000 population
Life expectancy: Total average 79.52 years, Male 76.18 years, Female 83.08 years
Official name: Kingdom of Spain/Espana, run by Parliamentary Monarchy
Chief of State: King Juan Carlos I (since 22nd November 1975),
Currency: Euro dollar (Euro €: Swiss Franc (CHF)= 1:1.5481) (20/10/2005)
GDP €846bn, real GDP growth 2.5% pa, GDP/head €27, 670
of which - agriculture 3.5%, industry 28.5%, services 68%.
Labour force: 19.33 million of which - agriculture 5.3%, manufacturing, mining and construction 30.1%, services 64.6% - Unemployment rate 10.4% total labour force
Budget: Revenues €383.7bn, Expenditures €386.4bn - Public debt 53.2% of GDP
National Holiday 12th October
Main cities (population): *Madrid* 3,016,000, *Barcelona* 1,527 000, *Seville* 704 000, *Valencia* 762 000, *Granada* 242 000
Airports: 156 (2004 est.)

Let us analyse some actual budget airline flights from the UK to Spain:-

---

[85] http://www.andalucia.com/spain/economy/home.htm

[86] http://www.odci.gov/cia/publications/factbook/geos/sp.html

Flight FR2638 London (Stansted) to Granada for one adult on Monday 19th December 2005 would cost 24.99 GBP 17:55-21:40 therefore 3hrs 45 minutes duration. FR2637 London (Stansted) to Granada for one adult on Tuesday 20th December 2005 would cost 39.99GBP 11:10-13:00 therefore 1hr 50minute duration. Price differential £15 between these two. These two flights are with Ryanair (ryanair.com)

However, Easyjet, flying to Barcelona on Monday 19th December 2005 would be as follows: flight #5131 London (Gatwick) to Barcelona 06:55-10:00 costs 19.99GBP. Flight #5135 London (Gatwick) to Barcelona 13:45-16:50 would cost 24.99GBP. Similar flights leaving Luton and Stansted cost 19.99GBP, therefore there would be a price differential of £20 from cheapest Easyjet flight to Barcelona to Ryanair flight FR2637 to Granada (easyjet.com).

Michael O'Leary, one of Ireland's richest men, has been Ryanair's CEO since 1994, transforming the company from small regional carrier into the most valuable airline in Europe. As of Monday June 06th this year, Ryanair had market capitalisation of €5bn euros ahead of Lufthansa at €4.7bn, British Airways €4.3bn, and Air France-KLM at €3.5bn. Market capitalisation is now four times higher than EasyJet at €1.3bn despite EasyJet having a higher turnover, similar passenger volumes and a slightly larger fleet. At the beginning of June 2005 Ryanair had increased pre-tax profit in the 12 month period to March 31st 2005 by 29.5%, meaning €295.9million profit[87].

Ryanair are currently in full support of Stansted airport building a second runway although Michael O'Leary condones BAA's monopoly of the three major airports Heathrow, Gatwick and Stansted. The cost is estimated to be £4bn for this expansion.

---

[87] Done, Kevin (Wednesday June 08th 2005:p24) FT – Aerospace Correspondent

The Green Dragon

Increased oil prices have meant it necessary to impose fuel surcharge on air tickets for all airlines, in response to which Ryanair shrugged off surging oil prices, reporting record annual profits. Their forecast for March 2006 includes traffic growth to rise from 23% to 27%, therefore 35million additional passengers; also, the J P Morgan profit estimates forecast for March 2006 for Ryanair will rise from €304m to €326m. Already, Ryanair's shares have closed 3.4% higher at €6.46. Average fares will drop down by 20% during the winter season. O'Leary's main aim being to step up passenger volumes to 70 million by the year 2012, thus making Ryanair Europe's largest airline by passenger numbers[88].

Air transport employs 4 million people, creating $400bn direct economic output. Therefore 4.5% global GDP is directly responsible to Air transport. This year's economy forecast growth will hold at 3.2%, though next year's forecast looks lower, falling to 2.8% (-0.4%). Spain remains one of the fastest growing economies in the Eurozone however, with real GDP 3.4% year-on-year.

Last year Spain posted a record €40bn Current Account deficit, equal to 5% GDP as imports bottomed and tourism declined as a direct consequence of the Madrid bombings on March 11th. According to the Chamber of Commerce, business confidence fell to its lowest level in two years in the first quarter of 2005, and is now expected to improve prospects of increase 15.3 points from 4.7 points in the first quarter 2006, boosted by lower oil prices. The US company Brent oil supplies Spain with oil at US$55/barrel. This is expected to drop to US$46.3/barrel in 2006.

Forecasts, assumptions and risks projected for the immediate future: i) Total employment will continue to grow; ii) the European Central Bank will cut interest rates late this year *and* in the first half of 2006 in reaction to weak Eurozone growth; iii)

---

[88] Done, Kevin (June 22nd/01st 2005:p22/p19) FT – Aerospace Correspondent

Oil prices and the Eurodollar value could appreciate more strongly than expected; iv) Further major terrorist assaults may occur; v) Equity markets fall back again; and vi) ECB fails to cut interest rates if Eurozones economic recovery continues to falter[89].vii) "Aviation emissions represent 15% of domestic emissions as at 2000. At present rates of growth that will become 66% by 2050" Friends of the Earth.

Both Ryanair and Easyjet are the current two leading UK low-cost airlines. New routes are continuously being established with a recent Easyjet expansion airway base being established at Euroairport Basel-Mulhouse-Freiburg, Switzerland. Matthew Garrahan writes that 27 million passengers have flown with Easyjet in the last 12 months, and that low-cost carriers have been experimenting with in-flight entertainments, economy class appeal, self-booking procedure and regional hubs[90].
Switzerland has at present 65 operating Airports.

EASYJET, founded March 1995, is now one of *Europe's* top 5 airlines in order of Lufthansa, Ryanair, Air France, BA and Easyjet (2 of which are low-cost carriers). Ray Webster (CEO Easyjet) proposed a merger, making a €584million offer to buy rival 'Go', and also purchased the option to acquire Deutsche-BA in next 12 months.

The Easyjet business model in a nutshell runs as: 1) simple fare structure offering a single fare at any one time for a specific flight ie value-for-money. 2) Unit costs maintaining high aircraft utilisation, no frills service, and focus on internet sales. 3) Strong branding. 4) Commitment to customer service. 5) Multi-base network high frequency point-to-point services on dense routes

---

[89] EBSCO e-journal 'Spain country monitor' September 2005
http://search.epnet.com/login.aspx?direct=true&db=buh&jid=50S

[90] Business Travel Special Report FT Mon Jun 13 2005 p1

The Green Dragon

within Europe. And 6) Strong corporate culture[91]. Given that, in theory, you could purchase an Easyjet ticket for £10, plus £5 passenger duty, paying £600 for BA economy class does not add up when you will arrive at the very same destination anyway!

Example routes from the UK to Switzerland could include the following: London (Gatwick) to Geneva, London (Luton) to Basel/Geneva, and London (Stansted) to Basel. Flight #2081 London (Luton) to Basel-Mulhouse on Monday 19th December 2005 would cost 29.99GBP 07:20-10.05, therefore 2hrs 45 minute duration. Flight #2085 London (Stansted) to Basel-Mulhouse also Monday 19th December 2005 would cost 49.99 GBP 13:05-15:45 therefore 2hrs 40 minute duration. Price differential £20 due to an afternoon start as opposed to early morning (easyjet.com).

The Swiss Confederation was born on 01st August 1291, since which time there has been a National Holiday every year on this date. UN member although EU neutral.
Chief of State: President and Head of Government Samuel Schmid (since 01/01/2005) *Population:* 7 489 370 (July 2005 est), *Population growth:* 0.49%
Area: (1,000sq km) 41.3
Major cities: (1,000 inhabitants) Zurich 355.3, Basel 180.0, Geneva 173.5, Bern 135.1
Birth rate: 9.77 births/1,000 population, *Death rate:* 8.48 deaths/1,000 population
Net migration: 3.58 migrants/1,000 population
Life expectancy: 80.39 years total, Male 77.58 years, Female 83.36 years
Languages: German 63.7%, French 20.4%, Italian 6.5%, Romansch 1.5%, Other 6%
Labour force: 3.77 million of which agriculture 4.6%, industry 26.3%, services 68.1%

---

[91] http://www.aci-europe.org/upload/144181672002aci%20july%202002%20all%20policy.pdf#search='easyjet%20ceo'

Reserves of foreign exchange and Gold 2003 $69.58bn, Public debt 57.2% GDP 2004
Budget: revenues $131.5bn – expenditures $140.4bn
Swiss Franc (CHF): Euro € = 1:0.6459 (20/10/2005)
GDP (ppp) 2004 $251.9bn, real growth rate 2004 1.8%, per capita 2004 $33,800
Unemployment rate 3.4% 2004
Agriculture: grains, fruits, vegetables, meat, eggs
Industry: machinery, chemicals, watches, textiles, precision instruments[92]

"Swiss Gold reserves per head outshine any other country. IN the year 2000 they started selling half of their 2600 tonnes to break the constitutional link between currency and metal. The Central Bank were to pass SwFr2.9bn (£1.3bn) to the state. Profits compromise operating earnings, complex back payments and SwFr400 million in gold related revenues"[93].

At a regional level we are looking at Basel and Zurich. Swiss regional languages include French in Geneva & Lausanne, German in Zurich, Basel & Bern, and Italian in Lugano. Romansch is usually spoken in the mountain regions only. The net economic benefits could be said to be chiefly touristic as depicted by the following:

Mediterranean Basel people have a great deal of savoir-vivre. Good food and drink are as important to them as art and culture. When museums and shops close their doors, Basel shows its more exuberant side. Young and old alike enjoy the lively nightlife. Basel Fasnacht Carnival is an annual 3 day event, providing maximum entertainment full of passions and creativity.

The Rhine is both a vital waterway and local place for recreation. The Rhine makes an important environmental and personal

---

[92] http://www.odci.gov/cia/publications/factbook/geos/sz.html

[93] FT (Tue December 07th 2004: p24) Haig Simonian

The Green Dragon

impact, contributing greatly to the high quality of life that Basel can offer its guests and residents.

Undulating hills of the Jura provide magnificent views and hiking/rambling paths abound. Laufenthal valley provides a rural idyll away from the hustle and bustle of city life. Skiing in winter is phenomenal with the mountains extremely accessible locally. Within an hour of Basel you can get to Zurich, Lucerne, Berne, Strasbourg, Colmar, or Freiburg im Breiggau[94].

The Zurich region contains pretty old towns, and the trendy new Zurich west district with glorious lake; Opera, ballet, theatre premieres, shows, musicals, art exhibitions in over 50 museums and 100 galleries. The famous Bahnhofstrasse and Limmatquai are a shoppers paradise. And over 1,700 restaurants and bars serve local and Swiss specialities ensuring nobody goes hungry[95].

Distribution and sales channels decreased levels of independent retailers giving way to a rise in self-service, discount stores and supermarkets. Retailers have setup organisations to provide wholesale purchasing, importing and other services. This vertical structure and centralized buying give them competitive advantage over independent retailers. There are over 150 franchises currently operating in the Swiss market, 25% of domestic origin, 25% American origin, and a large% French origin. Note companies such as Coca-Cola, Pepsi, Yopplait, and restaurants McDonalds, Burger King, Wendy's, Pizza Hut, and Subway to name but a few.

---

[94]

http://www.usa.myswitzerland.com/en/destinations.cfm?category=Destinations&subcat=Basel

[95]

http://www.usa.myswitzerland.com/en/destinations.cfm?category=Destinations&subcat=Zurich

Direct marketing home-shopping has become a greatly popular way of selling in Switzerland. Over 5,700 people are members of the Swiss Association of Direct Marketing companies (Schweizerischer Vernband der Direktverkauts-Fromen VDF) With over one million clients from 1998 meant that net worth would be now over SwFr283 million. Major products are sold in food and nutrition eg multivitamins, food supplements, power-drinks (containing vitamins, minerals, and proteins). Major competitors in Switzerland are: Nahrin AG, Edifors, NBC Nutrition, and Bodycare Concept AG.

Joint Ventures are classified as ordinary partnerships (Einfachnce Gesellschaft) in Switzerland, and licensing is absolutely essential to acquire know-how, adding value to imported raw goods and services. Advertising and trade promotion pronounces the highest density of newspapers in the world here, due to the variety of languages and cultural diversity within the nation. Over 100 daily/weekly newspapers are distributed for free.

Radio and TV: the Swiss Broadcasting Company (SRG) is the private, non-profit monopoly organization financed through compulsory listener/viewer fees. 9 radio stations in total…3 French, 3 German,and 3 Italian for each language region. Switzerland also possesses one of the best intellectual property protection regimes in the world right now[96].

Doing business in Switzerland has some most important ethics and etiquette associated, similar to other Northern European countries and the US eg formal, smart dress wear; use of family name rather than first name; punctuality being especially important in German-speaking areas; and setting appointment schedules as drop-ins are considered rude.

---

[96] BUSINESS SOURCE PREMIER - MARKETING AND DISTRIBUTION IN SWITZERLAND
SWITZERLAND ECONOMIC STUDIES (2000:P60)

Finally, the excellent business infrastructure in Switzerland also promotes these economic benefits: international airports at Zurich and Geneva, with smaller airports at Basel and Bern; roads, rail networks, urban public transport unsurpassed and telecommunications always modern, with deregulation causing a drop in prices[97].

So, having looked into the two European regions we should now consider the driving forces behind economic success. Why do people want to establish new airlines and bases around the world? The issue here, to me, is about entrepreneurship. Wickham defines entrepreneurship as "concerned with creating and managing vision and communicating that vision to other people. It is about demonstrating leadership, motivating people and being effective in getting people to accept change[98]."

Europe 2003, the Commission published a green paper on entrepreneurship. A new entrepreneurial agenda Action Plan was subsequently presented to the European spring council 2004, to the member states. The entrepreneurship action plan contains the following 5 strategic focuses:

i) changing the way society looks at entrepreneurs
ii) creating the conditions to encourage more people to become entrepreneurs.
iii) allowing SME's and entrepreneurs to play a full role in driving growth and enabling them to remain competitive.
iv) improving the financial flow to SMEs and entrepreneurs.
v) creating a more SME-friendly regulatory and administrative framework.

From these five focuses, *nine key actions* are to be performed to transform these five strategic objectives into concrete results.

---

[97] HISTORICAL BACKGROUND - SWITZERLAND ECONOMIC STUDIES (2000:p104)
http://search.epnet.com/login.aspx?direct=time&db=buh&an=5847937

[98] Chell Elizabeth (2001:pp28/29) Entrepreneurship: globalisation, innovation and development – Thomson Learning

The Commission has defined with member states these 'key actions'[99]:

Key Action#1- fostering entrepreneurial mindsets through school education to promote entrepreneurship on a European and national level.
Key Action#2-reducing the stigma of failure
Key Action#3-facilitating the transfer of businesses strives to foster the development of marketplaces.
Key Action#4-improving social security of small business owners focuses on reviewing current states of social security for small owners.
Key Action#5-tailor-made support for women and ethnic minorities.
Key Action#6A-facilitating SMEs business cooperation in internal market
Key Action#6B-fostering innovative clusters
Key Action#7-more equity and stronger balance sheets
Key Action#8-listening to SMEs promotes policy-makers and stakeholders in the policymaking process at EU level
Key Action#9-simplification of tax compliance. Simplify and reduce tax compliance procedures for SMEs.

In evaluation overall we could say that of all the regions discussed, Catalunia would be the major *industrial* region of those selected thriving from the likes of Barcelona, whilst Andalucia is largely *tourist* orientated thriving from Granada and Sevilla. In Switzerland the selected regions Basel and Zurich in the North thrive also from tourism, but being a land-locked country, significant interest comes from the North, from Germany and Austria in particular to these two regions. Interestingly the two chosen countries are rather more separate than many other European nations.

---

[99] The Journal of the Local Economy policy unit vol20 #1 (Feb 2005:pp99-101) The Green paper on entrepreneurship - Sonia Herrero-Rada.

The Green Dragon

As for the budget airlines, Ryanair has the edge now over Easyjet and continues to improve with O'Leary setting newer, bigger goals all the time. Ray Webster is not complacent though at all and continues to improve the Easyjet service on a daily basis. All in all, if you are flying within Europe you can't go wrong with either of these two airlines, value-for-money and good time-keeping. You will get there!

Bibliography

- BUSINESS SOURCE PREMIER

1) http://search.epnet.com/login.aspx?direct=true&db=buh&an=58 47936 'Cultural and Demographic risks in Switzerland' Switzerland Economic Studies 2000 p93

2) ~ ~ ~ ~ ~ ~ ~ ~
=5847932 'Marketing and Distribution in Switzerland' Switzerland Economic Studies 2000 p60

3) ~ ~ ~ ~ ~ ~ ~ ~
=5847937 'Historical background' Switzerland Economic Studies 2000 p104

- Chell, Elizabeth (2001) Entrepreneurship: Globalization, innovation and development – Thomson learning
- Click R W, Coval J D (2002) The theory and practice of International Financial Management – Prentice Hall
- Done, Kevin (June 01/06/08/22 2005) The Financial Times 'aerospace correspondent'
- e-journal Spain Country Monitor (Sep 2005) EBSCO
- Financial Times (Jun 14 2005) Special Report ' Spain'
- Garrahan, Matthew (Mon Jun 13 2005) Financial Times Business Travel Special Report
- Harrison, Joseph (1978) An economic history of modern Spain – Manchester University Press
- Herrero-Rada, Sonia (Feb 2005) The Journal of the Local Economy Policy Unit - Vol 20 #1 'The Green Paper on Entrepreneurship'
- http://www.andalucia .com/spain/economy/home.html
- http://search.epnet.com/login.aspx?direct=true&db=buh&jid=50S
- http://usa.myswitzerland.com/en/destinations.cfm?category=Destinations&subcat=Zurich
- http://www.odci.gov/cia/publications/factbook/geos/sz.html
- http://www.odci.gov/cia/publications/factbook/geos/sp.html

- Journal of Economic Policy 39- July 2004 : Blackwell – Engel & Rogers *"Euro's price dispersion"*
- Kirby, David A (2003) Entrepreneurship – McGraw Hill
- Lieberman, Sima (1982) The contemporary Spanish economy: A historical perspective – George Allen & Unwin
- Lynskey & Yonekura (2002) Entrepreneurship & Organization – OUP
- OECD ECONOMIC SURVEYS SWITZERLAND 1995 & (JULY)1996
- Parker, Geoffrey (1994:ch12 p170) *Contemporary International Relations : a guide to theory.* Printer Publishers London New York ----- *GEOPOLITIK coined by Swedish political scientist Rudolf Kjellen University of Gothenburg – the spatial study of relationships among states and the implications of these relationships for the morphology of the political map as a whole.
- Roman, Manuel (1997) Growth and Stagnation of the Spanish Economy – Avebury
- Salmon, Keith (1995) *The Modern Spanish Economy : transformation & integration into Europe* 2nd edition– Pinter
- Schweizeizersche NationalBank Geld, Wahrung und konjunkur (September 1997) Bulletin #3, and (December 1997) Bulletin #4.
- Simonian, Haig (Dec 07 2004:p24) The Financial Times
- Wright, Alison (1977) The Spanish Economy 1959-1076 – MacMillan Press ltd

Appendix 9 - Strategic Management
26390

"Stakeholders are those individuals or groups who depend on the organisation to fulfil their own goals and on whom, in turn, the organisation depends". (Johnson & Scholes p179)

Using examples where appropriate, discuss how the strategy of an organisation might be affected if/when stakeholders pursue their own objectives.

Module Leader: Steve Braund
Due for: Thursday, 23rd February 2006

Appendix 9 – Introduction

The International Olympic Committee (IOC) was founded June 23rd, 1894 by the French educationalist Baron Pierre de Coubertin, who had the idea of reviving the Olympic Games of Ancient Greece. Although at the time the man met head on with immense cynicism, disbelief and indifference his vision of "all sports for all people" proved to be a winner in the long term as we now are able to appreciate today. The five Olympic values universal to all are: sportsmanship, education, exceeding ones expectations, solidarity, peace and happiness[100]. We could think of these values as strategies, and stakeholders as adopting these as objectives. How would a change of objectives affect the organisation and the stakeholders?

"Strategy is the direction and scope of an organisation over the long term, which achieves advantage in a changing environment through its configuration of resources and competency with the aim of fulfilling stakeholder expectations[101]".

In this case, we could consider stakeholders to include competitive athletes, fans and supporters, coaches, media representatives, the executive board and organising committee. We will relate these stakeholders to many potential objectives and how they would inter-relate and change as a consequence of objective shifts. Are the two absolutely co-dependent? Are they cooperative, collaborative, or conflictive? Or are they so rigid in their consequence that the slightest change in any one policy will cancel all related activity? These possibilities will be studied in greater depth throughout.

This essay will *describe* values in terms of strategies and potential consequences of a change in objectives. We will

---

[100] www.olympic.org/uk/index_uk.asp

[101] Johnson, Scholes, Whittington (2005:9) Exploring Corporate Strategy 7th edition

identify specific organisational strategies and examine the associated rapport with the stakeholder parties. Strategies and values are to be highlighted along with examples of academic theory to demonstrate the meaning in a wider context. Various hypotheses shall be presented and their outlook postulated upon. Following which I will *discuss* internal strengths and weaknesses of the organisation, and consider external opportunities and threats too. The evaluation will appraise the given material, the summary will exhibit what I have covered, and the conclusion will present my findings.

Describe
The five universal Olympic values are: sportsmanship, education, exceeding ones expectations, solidarity, peace and happiness. These five values represent the very reason that athletes devote their lives and make such sacrifice towards their objectives. The Olympics represents an ideal towards which people stand up for and live with passion. The Olympic spirit is kept alive by these five values created by IOC. Sport, culture and respect present the three pillars of the Olympic ideal.

In terms of stakeholder objectives we will take each value and regard some related possibilities. *Sportsmanship* encourages each athlete with an absolute obligation to give better than their best, to strive beyond all known achievement, to not only win the race but, at the same time be graceful in the face of defeat and accept that participation in this race means experience necessary to gain the edge in the next. Sportsmanship means knowing how to win even when somebody else is winning. *Education* is constant and never ending; we are always improving, always learning, always evolving, often without realising. We are continuously becoming and in doing so we are educating others too. *Exceeding ones expectations* in life gives us a huge survival guidance. We are either living or dying, building or destroying, creating or destructing. If we do not build then we die, no matter what the context. We are designed to innovate and by continuously building a new level every day we are thus exceeding our expectations. *Solidarity* translates as unity in diversity. The whole world comes together for 17 days at a time to celebrate pure achievement. Everybody unites over the Olympics (courtesy of IOC organisation and competitive stakeholder participants). P*eace and happiness* come from fulfilling lifetime objectives having come through all manner of challenge on the journey. We are called to achieve certain objectives and in this case, those who achieve Olympic Gold would surely experience profound peace and happiness. "Higher, faster, stronger!" Athletes *intend* to win the gold, supporters intend to *see* the athletes win the gold, and the organisers intend to *enable* the athletes to win the gold.

Looking ahead we can anticipate the Beijing Summer Olympics 2008, Vancouver Winter Games 2010 and London Summer Games 2012. Currently in the Turin Winter Games 2006 Shelly Rudman (UK) developed an objective to win Gold, having begun skeleton run just 40 months previously. She is Olympic silver medallist now and no doubt maintains her stakeholder objective[102]. The organisation is able to confer universal strategy for every stakeholder who determines to participate. Steve Redgrave (UK) 5 times Olympic Rowing Gold medallist Athens 2004, Sydney 2000, Atlanta 1996, Barcelona 1992, Seoul 1988, as stakeholder in the IOC has changed objectives now from himself winning gold to coaching other stakeholder candidates to achieve the same objective. Rhona Martin (UK) and her curling team came out with Olympic Gold at the 2002 Salt Lake City Winter Games. This stakeholder objective remained the same 4 years later at Turin 2006, although the result has proved to be different. Likewise, David Murdoch and the GB men's curling team came to Turin this month with Golden objectives only to have to reevaluate for next time.

Identify
Michael Payne (stakeholder - media journalist) has developed eight objectives by which he perceives the development for the

---

[102] Mackay D (17/02/06) Rudman strikes Silver to warm Britain'sHearts – Guardian Newspaper

Beijing Summer Olympics 2008[103]. 1) Leadership sets the pace (regarding especially Juan Antonio Samaranch transforming the Olympic movement from a floundering cottage industry around 1980 to the most lucrative sporting event in the entire world today), 2) The starting line is the bottom line (we all begin where we begin, each level to be developed, each step to be taken), 3) Only do deals you can live with (optimism yes, but with account of current reality to build from. Risk taking to be measured not to be ignored), 4) Zero tolerance – sorry doesn't work (if you are responsible for making a mistake then you must be fully prepared to take the consequences associated with the mistake), 5) Hold the torch aloft (never take your eyes off from the flame, let the whole world bear witness), 6) Manage the grey areas (improve on what needs improving, get your hands dirty where necessary, clear up, stand up, be counted), 7) Fast reflexes, using trauma as a catalyst (take the lessons you learn from disaster as a point of learning, do not be offset by immediate traumas), 8) Appeal to the highest common denominator (make win/win situations for all, there must be universal attraction in order for the system to operate at the standard expected).

In terms of academic theory, where stakeholders change their objectives the organisation must be adaptable in strategy, instantly able to anticipate that stakeholder objectives *will* change par for the course. The external environment presents us with contingency theories, organisational ecology, and industrial organisation. The internal environment equates to Resource Based View[104]. Contingency theory (i) identifies structural mechanisms and operating methods that ensure long-term survival of firms in different kinds of settings (Burns and Stalker 1961). Coping with uncertainty is identified as the essence of

---

[103] Payne M (Spring 2005) Reinventing the rings – insights into Global Business : Business Strategy Review Vol 16 Issue # 1

[104] Guruw R V, Post J E, Berger P D (Autumn 2005:86) Adapt or adapt – lessons for strategy : Journal of General Management Vol 31 Issue #1

the adaptation process and 'co-alignment' of technology, task environment, organisational design and structure postulated to be necessary to deal with the uncertainty (Thompson 1967). Population ecologists (ii) advocate Darwinian principles of survival and natural selection combined with neo-institutionalists shaping organisational choices by cultural-institutional roles. Both perspectives converge relating adaptability of an organisation to its ability to learn and perform consistent with changing environmental contingencies alone. Industrial organisation (ii) achieves congruence between internal Strengths and Weaknesses of the firm, and external Opportunities and Threats in the environment. We will discuss this specific area at a later stage. Embedded in the neoclassical economic theory, the IO paradigm postulates that the structure of the industry influences the conduct of the firm and this in turn determines its performance. Resource Based View (iv) alerts us to the need to distinguish successful firms from others based on certain unique, inimitable resource endowments or capabilities that the former possess, which enable them to adapt better to changes in the environment.

Discuss

The Beijing Games 2008 will cost over $40bn (£22.9bn) and over 10,500 athletes from more than 202 nations will be present. It is expected that 20,200 media representatives will be working as journalists to record the event in every detail which for China this means that in just 17 days, more journalists will visit the country than in the entire past 100 years. The phenomenal growth over the last 20 years has seen a cottage industry grow from the 1980 Moscow Games in a financial abyss, to a multi-billion dollar global success, making and breaking media empires, launching and reinvigorating global brands, whilst bringing investment across otherwise distant borders between nations[105].

---

[105] Payne M (Spring 2005) Reinventing..... ~ ~ ~
~ ~ ~ ~

Internal strengths – Passion ignites great momentum with the power of the Gold objective presenting such enthusiasm and strength by association with the Olympic ideal. . Now presided by Jacques Rogge the 8th IOC President elected 16th July 2001, taking over the reins from Juan Antonio Samaranch (Spanish Honorary President for life) inducted in the CIO 1966. Samaranch being responsible for the 1980-2001 IOC economic turnaround seeing $200 000 (£114, 317) become $40bn (£22.9bn) within 25 years. "Olympism is a philosophy of life, exaltation and combining in a balanced whole the qualities of body, will and mind. Blending sport with culture and education, olympism seeks to create a way of life based on the joy found in effort, the education, value of and example and respect for universal fundamental ethical principles[106]".

Internal weaknesses – Turin Winter Games 2006 exhibits a blood doping scandal in the Austrian biathlon/cross-country skiing team. Members discovered with 100s syringes for blood analysis, distilled water in vials, antidepressants, asthma medication and consequently exposed as allegations of potential blood-doping to enhance performance. Testing for erythropoietin (EPO) a listed banned substance will take several days[107]. Candidate host cities who receive rejection (most) may experience turbulent times as their people go through bitter disappointment for a certain period of time. For 2012 there were 9 host candidates: Istanbul, Leipzig, London, Paris, New York, Rio de Janeiro, Havana, Moscow and Madrid. During the lengthy construction period of the Olympic village, local residents would feel disturbed at times by the constant commotion associated with creating the village.

---

[106] www.olympic.org/uk/organisation/missions/charter_uk.asp
Olympic Charter fundamental principles paragraph 2

[107] Popham P (22/02/06) *A drug raid, a car chase and a scandal on an Olympic scale* : The Independent Newspaper Olympic Sports

External opportunities – the media get to have a field day with journalists employed on a vast scale to monitor every little detail caused by the IOC's organizational objectives. National pride springs up from being appointed the host of an Olympic games, enabling profitable capitalisation to occur in direct association with the Games. Sponsors gain advantageous publicity in relation to excellence of achievement. Political Relations between nations have potential for significant cooperation as integrity comes forth. Even with just one representative from a nation, this fact looks great for a country and so existing potentially improves an entire reputation forthwith.

External threats – Police intervention in Turin this month with the Austrian biathlon/cross-country skiing team, caused Walter Mayer (Coach) to drive through a barrier on being chased by Italian Police, having been banned by the IOC for a blood doping scandal at the 2002 Salt Lake City Winter Games. The IOC must reevaluate the situation because of this stakeholder activity. 1980 US and 1984 USSR Games saw both countries opting to boycott the others Olympics in turn as a declaration of intent during the Cold War (used as a political pawn). Language barriers for such a multi-national event require translators, interpreters and linguists, employable to ensure complete communication for all. Creed and culture present very real external threats for the IOC and stakeholders. The IOC has complete responsibility to fully accommodate, cater for and be hospitable to all visitors within the Olympic village.

Evaluation

We have described, identified and discussed various stakeholder and organizational strategies in context of the IOC. The effects of change have been taken into consideration were the stakeholder to pursue their own objectives. In so doing it could be said that:

A) Stakeholders depend on the organisation to fulfil their own goal as individuals and as groups. Athletes aiming for Olympic gold rely on the IOC to create the tournament. IOC committee stakeholders rely on the organisation to gain sufficient publicity, advertising, marketing, media attention in order to attract maximum investment to support the event. Coaches rely on athletes, not so much the organisation, although were in not for the IOC this particular tournament would not exist, even though World/European/National/Regional championship tournaments would still go ahead on similar prerogative.

B) The organisation relies on the stakeholders to fulfil its goals. The IOC would never have a purpose were it not for the presence and continuous influence of the stakeholder members. I feel that in this case the organisation is much more dependent on the stakeholders as a survival mechanism than the stakeholders are on the organisation. It would be easy enough for stakeholders to switch and focus their attentions on other tournaments, whereas the IOC would not be capable of operating even for one minute without the loyalty, commitment and dedication of the stakeholder members.

Summary
The International Olympic Committee (IOC) represents the organisation, the contenders, fans, coaches, supporters, executive board, media, and organisers represent the stakeholders. Sportsmanship, education, exceeding ones own expectations, solidarity, peace and happiness represent the primary strategy and the stakeholders' objective revolves around winning Gold. With this in mind, any change in stakeholder objective would be unusual here, although many contenders would accept that they need to develop more strongly for the next time. Strategies in this case are highly collaborative with stakeholder change resulting in organisational changes and vice versa, for example the strategy where to locate the next Games? This reality affects everybody.

Payne's Beijing strategies provide us with a view point from the organisation's perspective, whilst the academic theory provides us with substance to confirm this relationship. Wright presents us with some very practical strategies from a professional management position. Internal strengths range from the Samaranch leadership to the all encompassing philosophy of

Olympism. Internal weaknesses include the Austrian Turin doping allegations and its repercussions for IOC, and candidate host city rejection. External opportunities revolve in favour of media attentions, political relations and favourable sponsorship. External threats again involve the Turin 2006 Austrian case and the effects of police allegations. Physically creating the Olympic village is such a threat to local residents.

Conclusion
The IOC as an organisation is more relient on its stakeholders to fulfil its goals than they are on the organisation. A change of stakeholder objectives would only encourage the organisation to review its strategies as course for continuous evaluation and improvement. Stakeholders do rely on the organisation to allocate specific tickets, provide refreshments, accommodations, memorabilia, entertainments, directions, and value experience. The people have the power to make or break an entire tournament. This is exactly the reason why the IOC will go out of their way to cater for every possible eventuality in anticipation of the event itself. The IOC need to maintain a strategy to ensure that the Games are complete, fully supported and all tickets sold.

Bibliography

Books

Johnson G & Scholes K (2002) *Exploring Corporate Strategy 6th edition* : FT Prentice Hall

Johnson G, Scholes K, Whittington R (2005) *Exploring Corporate Strategy 7th editions - Text and Cases* : FT Prentice Hall

Joyce P & Woods A (2001) Strategic Management – *a fresh approach to developing skills, knowledge and creativity* : MBA Kogan Page

Journals

Beer M & Eisenstat R A (2004:82-89) *How to have an honest conversation about your business strategy :* Harvard Business Review February 2004

Gavetti G & Rivkin J W (2005) *How strategists really think – tapping the power of analogy* : Harvard Business Review April 2005

Guruw R V, Post J E, Berger PD (2005:83-106) *Adapt or adapt – lessons for strategy* : Journal of General Management Autumn 2005 Vol 31 Issue#1

McGrath R G & MacMillan I C (2005:80-89) *Market busting growth – strategies for exceptional business* : Harvard Business Review March 2005

Ozbilgin M & Penno M (2005:920-932) *Corporate disclosure and operational strategy 'finance Vs operational success'* : Management Science June 2005 Vol 51 Issue # 6

Payne, M (2005) *Reinventing the Rings – insights into global business* : Business Strategy Review Spring 2005 Vol 16 Issue#1

Wright R P (2004:61-78) *Top manager's strategic cognitions of the strategy making process: differences between high and low performing firms* : Journal of General Management Autumn 2004 Vol 30 Issue # 1

ejournals/ IOC websites

Baum J R & Wally S (2003) *Strategic decision speed and firm performance* : Strategic Management Journal November 2003

Vol 24 Issue # 11 (Proquest: http://proquest.umi.com/pqdweb?index=4&did=530914211&SrchMode=34sid=21Fmt=3&VInst=PROD&VType=PQD&RQT=309&VName=PQD&TS=1140295621&clientId=25727&aid=1)
www.olympic.org/uk/index_uk.asp
www.olympic.org/uk/organisation/missions/charter_uk.asp

Newspapers
Mackay D (Friday, 17th February 2006) *Rudman strikes Silver to warm Britain's hearts* : The Guardian Newspaper Olympic Sports
Popham P (Wednesday, 22nd February 2006) *A drug raid, a car chase and a scandal on an Olympic scale* : The Independent Newspaper Olympic Sports

Appendix 10 - Table of Contents

1.0) Cover Page

2.0) Table of Contents

3.0) Executive Summary

4.0) Business Proposal

5.0) Letter of Transmittal

6.0) Introduction with aims, objectives and mission statement

7.0) SWOT Analysis using sub-categories: professional, practical, personal, environmental, financial, initiative, and Rationale

8.0) Financial projections – Regular incomes/outgoings, expected turnovers, special service charges, product itemisation, customer base.

9.0) Research methodology, findings, and analysis – project limitations, questionnaire design, Quasar motives.

10.0) Conclusions and recommendations

11.0) Reference section

12.0) Appendices: A1 Costa Coffee Initiatives
A2 Quasar Managerial Approach
A3 Weekly Schedule

A4 Listed Café Respondents
A5 Sample Questionnaire

A6 Disclaimer

The Green Dragon

Quasar Coffee Shop

Presented to: Professor Harness
Module: Independent Study
Code: 26432
Deadline: Tuesday, 28th March 2006

© Quasar Coffee Shop March 2006

Executive Summary

This project follows the premise of setting up a new coffee shop venture in the local neighbourhood in the name of Quasar Coffee Shop. The business proposal overleaf gives location and contact details, whilst the letter of transmittal goes into greater depth about the whole study.

- Introduction provides some background context to the proposal and sets the format of the report with aims, objectives plus the Quasar mission statement. The whole document is interspersed with constructive quotes from respondents regarding their own views on coffee shops; Essential for nurturing any new venture.

- SWOT analysis regards internal strengths/weaknesses, and external threats/ opportunities affecting Quasar from the neighbourhood. Subdivisions categorise into professional, practical, personal, environmental, financial, initiative. These provide specific examples to support each case. Rationale also provides support here.

- Financial projections are based on existing figures, so regular incomes/outgoings and predicted profits represent actuality. Special service charges also included for trades personnel, and other overheads besides refreshments. Calculations are as accurate as possible – customer base represents best – worst scenarios.

- Research methodology stems from theories, relevant to this topic – Quasar is a sole trader, motives are aired here. Limitations also present themselves, largely in the form of misrepresentation, defamation, or non-response. Questionnaire structure is considered, as are the five steps to venture establishment.

- Conclusions cover the SWOT findings, along with finances needed. Recommendations make referral to continuation with gaining knowledge about the coffee trade, especially to develop specialist skills in time.

- References from books, journals, periodicals demonstrate research, whilst appendices demonstrate Costa Coffee initiative, Quasar management style, Weekly rota, Coffee shops visited with surveys, example questionnaire, and official disclaimer.

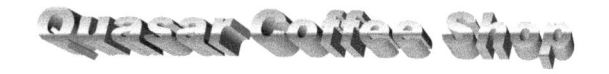

Quasar Coffee Shop

Address:
105 Cottingham Road,
Hull,
E Yorks,
HU5 2DH

Phone: (01482) 445588
E-mail: jk@quasarcoffee.co.uk
Website: www.quasarcoffee.co.uk

Manager/Owner: Jamie Kershaw
Baristas: Donna Wilkinson
Steve Morgan
      Bethany Thompson
      Anna Cuthbertson
      William Jones

Quasar Coffee Shop is a cafeteria for all to enjoy. Whether you are looking to sit quietly and read a newspaper whilst enjoying a unique coffee taste sensation, or to share the experience with friends whilst appreciating live music and poetry, there are moments for all.

We offer an unrivalled quality and variety of food and beverages at cutting edge prices, and our doors are open for you from 7am - 11pm Monday – Friday, 8am – 8pm weekends.

Letter of Transmittal

Jamie Kershaw,

Quasar Coffee Shop,

105 Cottingham Road,

Hull,

E Yorks,

HU5 2DH

Tuesday, 28th March 2006

Dear Professor Harness,

The following project has been written in the format of: Introduction with aims, objectives and mission statement, SWOT analysis–subheadings: professional, practical, personal, environmental, financial, initiative. Rationale follows to support the basis for these beliefs, then Financial Projections, Research Methodology, findings and analysis, Limitations of Study, Conclusions with Recommendations, References, and finally Appendices. Marketing to specific target groups, methods of advertising Quasar, and practicalities of constructing the cafeteria will be scrutinized.

Financial projections shall be forecast in the form of expected regular incomes and expenditures, specific product itemisation, staff costs, lease of property, supply costs, advertising costs, and other accountable profits-payments.

Research included in this project has come largely from two forms. Existing local coffee shops (staff surveys), and more academic research regarding the coffee trade: on-line, journals plus periodical articles, relevant text book passages, and word of mouth. Clients have been willing to provide their opinions on necessary skills useful in the trade along with gaps presenting need for development. Opinions on associated risks with starting up a small business venture also contribute towards building a more complete picture.

The main challenges I faced in writing this report have stemmed from making personal visits to local coffee shops in Hull, York and Beverley, and attempting to elicit specific company details from employees within the business whilst completing my questionnaires. Many cafes felt unwilling to provide their financial data on account of security issues. I required a letter stating the confidentiality of the project from yourself (Professor Harness) in order for some café managers to be willing to elaborate a little more about their coffee shop. Persuasion skills were put to the test in order to attract somebody to spend their time answering questions for my project, rather than earning. A certain pressure developed en route too. Most cafes which I approached proved happy and willing to divulge a little information for this purpose although certain outright rejections also occurred. Converting the given information from the questionnaires and from the sources of academic research has enabled more meaningful information for the report. I have organised the report like so as I believe this format to be convenient to read through and logically sequential.

Recommendations for further study would include the option of designing surveys for other groups of client (especially customers) – how would you improve the coffee shop? What developments would you support? Do you agree with the prices? What incentives would attract you to remain loyal to this café? What defining factor would make you want to remain in association with this one business? For a project of this size it has been possible only to regard the selected group, a more complete report would require at least double the amount of words available.

                                                Yours sincerely,

Jamie Kershaw
Quasar Coffee Shop Owner/Manager
(01482) 445588
jk@quasarcoffee.co.uk

Introduction

This project provides a projection of ideas on the premise of founding a new coffee shop venture. Based on grass roots research, word of mouth advice from baristas, and supported by substantial academic findings the report will include a detailed SWOT analysis – professional, practical, personal, environmental, financial, initiative. Marketing considerations along with suggestions for development from alternative viewpoints have developed from my academic research which has taken place in Hull, York and Beverley. More than 25 coffee shops were approached of which most have been willing to provide a significant response for this project (see appendices for example questionnaire [5], for listed respondents [4], and for letter of disclosure [6]).

For UK based coffee shops the vast majority of supplies come from Africa, Asia, or S & C America. Countries such as Nicaragua, Peru, Brazil, Guatemala and Colombia export their coffee to the UK providing Fair Trade coffee in our cafeterias, which enables benefits to the local farmers and their home communities. In this way, the UK plays a *critical* role in global relations because of providing coffee supplied from plantations worldwide. The cause is supported.

The aims and objectives of Quasar coffee shop can be defined with the assistance of a unique, self-fulfilling mission statement:-

"A continuous provision of excellent quality food and beverages for the community which we serve with humour, gratitude and pride towards our customers" (2006)

In terms of this report we will learn about the underlying theory representing a foundation for the development of practical working premises at an opportune time in the future. The five stages of new venture appraisal will be highlighted within the conclusion, stage one of which involves research as portrayed in this project.

"Don't copy others, stick to what you are good at. Create your own niche and stick at it...do not reinvent the wheel!" (Café One Newland Avenue 2005)

SWOT Analysis[108]

The following analysis indicates useful existing skill sets, current gaps for development, opportunities and threats surrounding Quasar Coffee Shop.

"Products are not just for coffee aficionados, but for everyone. We try to meet all needs. Good location, reasonable prices and the best coffee around" (Starbucks Coffee House: Borders book store ~ York city (2005).

Internal Strengths identified by the professionals:
Professional Number One ~ Passion for coffee! Each barista should demonstrate the ability to work quickly and logically thinking quickly on their feet whilst maintaining professional standards. Fitness should prove adequate for the job, multi-tasking with pride of presentation, commitment to the job, organizational skills, taking time for customers as real people and not merely a number on a seat. Knowledge of the coffee market (suppliers, labour laws, Fairtrade, tax regimes) and technical equipment instils confidence when questions arise. Careful management of people/ stock/ furnishings, and availability of trade skills for maintenance (eg plumbing, electrician, decorator) would build more professional appeal for Quasar.

Practical features that would benefit the café could include wheelchair access with assistance if required, specific tailoring to dietary requirement eg organic, vegetarian, gluten-free, vegan or labels for allergies printed on products; Provision of teacakes and handmade cakes for elderly people, milkshakes for younger

---

[108] All SWOT research taken from Hull, York, Beverley coffee shops. See Appendix 4 for listings: completed questionnaires available on request (November 2005 – March 2006).

people or children, and non-dairy soya milk for those who request. Culinary skills amongst staff along with optimum consideration for health, hygiene and personal cleanliness to keep the preparation areas germ-free are essential. Knowledge of product/service being provided and understanding customer needs permit an array of different preferences to be managed. Comfort levels can be facilitated with bean bags, sofas, divans, armchairs, rugs, interesting display art/decor, background music and display of various flora/fauna entities. Tropical fish in a tank are often displayed.

"Café Nero is a contemporary Italian style coffee house with a neighbourhood feel. We have room for pushchairs/babychanging facilities, comfy seats for individuals & groups. We follow the six service steps for maximum efficiency" (Beverley 2005)

Personal skills prove all important in business ie customer oriented, friendly disposition, sense of humour, good communication skills, diplomacy; dealing with all types of people in a friendly way, offering babychanging facilities and having the memory capacity to recall names, faces, interests, family situations et al demonstrate competence in coping with pressure. Being able to cope with small details aka 'Hawk Eye', making fast snap decisions, demonstrating outgoing persona with entrepreneurial flair are strengths. Adaptability to change, perseverance, and willingness to take risks are key characteristics for developing barista charisma.

"Response to customer needs is directly related to the make up of the customers who come in." (Planet Coffee Newland Avenue 2006)

Environmental strengths would include the display of health/ hygiene/ security and catering qualification certificates allowing clients to appreciate the stance of the café. Meticulous standards of hygiene and the maintenance of a comfortably warm venue provide customers with a favourable situation to appreciate for a while.

Financial ability to set fair prices and pay bills on schedule, to deal reliably with finances at all times and demonstrate astute accounting skills would enable Quasar to make optimum investments in friendly baristas, quality beverages, tasty foodstuffs, and up-to-date equipment. Negotiating skills for supplier bartering can represent significant deals if the timing is right.

Initiative in forwards-thinking can be constantly encouraged: "What else can we offer the customer? Which situations should we anticipate and prepare for?" A proactive teamwork spirit amongst staff apparent to customers would assist in providing incentives and a unique atmosphere within the cafeteria. Internet access also represents opportunity here. Employment of international students is said to improve this sense of diversity. The above selection of strengths would contribute to mutually represent a company's reputation. See Appendix 1 for Costa Coffee Initiatives.

"Love for coffee and love for service."(Lemon Tree: York station 2005)
"The best espresso this side of Milan!" (Café Nero, York City 2005)
"Being the best at what we do." (Gingers, Beverley 2005)

Internal Weaknesses identified within the same six categories as follows:

Professional lack of ownership experience would be main weakness in this venture.

Practical flaws would stem from lack of sufficient client base, being situated in a bad location such as inaccessible or unapparent to passers-by, keeping produce fresh is an absolute obligation - an expectation! We would aspire to maintain customer interest in the business, ensuring a good product base, employing the most able staff.

Personal weaknesses would involve lack of charisma, being flat, boring, fatigued, shabby in appearance, disassociated from the job in hand (unprofessional), thinking only 'what is in this for me?' rather than taking others and wider issues into consideration. Personal conflicts would also disturb the working internal atmosphere.

Environmentally smoking would be the prominent issue here. Plenty of non-smokers enjoy visiting cafes for refreshments, therefore a smoky environment would be unfavourable and conflict with maintaining hygiene standards within the business.

Financial weakness would stem from generating income from scratch, not having sufficient income to break-even, finding the best value suppliers via logistics operations, and the uncertainty of being able to gain corporate sponsors presenting significant challenge for Quasar, always risking loss of money.

Initiative weakness is only weakness if you view failure as an end in itself not a stepping stone towards learning new successful means. Building a credible reputation from scratch takes initiative and requires constant creative contribution in order to maintain customer interest.

"We look at our service – how we can give a better service, ways to speed up the service but be friendly. Always forward thinking – about what else we can offer the customer." (Continental café Student Union HUU 2005)

External Opportunities represent how Quasar could best be marketed and developed.

Professional radio broadcasting, local media publicity through newspaper/magazine circulation, and distribution of posters/flyers around the neighbourhood enhance credibility for Quasar Coffee Shop.

Practical advantages begin with fair trade and organic products available for sale on-site to attract like-minded consumers, plus provision of an on-site bakery to make fresh produce every day simultaneously creating alluring aromas for the café. Niche market opportunities along with product placement, attract specialist tastes. Facilities inviting performers on talent nights such as music, comedy, or poetry readings; coffee cards offer transferable 'points' to accumulate and redeem for a free drink or food item could ensure a loyal customer base.

"Being unique in having our own style of continental, international cuisine whilst keeping standards at a very high level" (Latitude Newland Avenue Hull 2006).

Personal word-of-mouth advertising spreads credibility, plus confirmation of consistently excellent produce heightens Quasar's reputation. Target Market for Quasar could be said to include: lovers of coffee - students, professionals, young or old, male and female. Reputation wins clients by delivery of quality promise.

Financial opportunity depends entirely on clients and sponsors coming forwards to offer their support to the enterprise. Suppliers or larger chains may also contribute.

*Initiative*s in the form of Promotions, Promotions, Promotions! Scholarship programs could be made available exclusively for current employees to study at university whilst working for the café (NB Canadian coffee chain Tim Hortons inc. currently employ this scheme[109]). Tim Hortons also offers a promotion known as 'R-r-roll up the rim' whereby customers can win anything from a chocolate chip cookie to CAD$1,000 cash, or a giant flat-screen TV system by simply unrolling the rim of the cup and revealing the message. We would be opportunists to develop a similar initiative here in the UK.

"Café Rouge was one of the UK's original café/bar concepts providing traditional French atmosphere/products/dishes/ service" (Café Rouge York 2005).
Stock rotation permits the regular incorporation of updated menus. A Café Latte could be served small, regular, or large with or without milk, cream, sugar, sweetener, flavoured syrup or a 99 flake. Thirdly, a suggestion box could be operated for customer feedback, complaints & compliments thereby allowing for future development to occur in the cafeteria as a consequence of suggestions given.

---

[109] http://www.timhortons.com/en/join/scholarship.html

"Consolidate on what you do best; get quality, quantity and price correct and cross your fingers."(Turpins coffee house Beverley 2005)

External Threats demonstrate pressures affecting Quasar and associates:
Professional contention presented from major Corporate conglomerate competitors such as Costa Coffee, Starbuck's, Café Nero, or Café Rouge automatically overshadow any smaller business starting out, although in more specific context, location is crucial, as is customer preference – many people enjoy exploring new territory with associated experience.
Practically location constitutes major responsibility for customer retention on account of accessibility. Property/equipment damage such as flooding, electrical faults, woodworm, broken windows, graffiti etc would be an unforeseen expense beyond the immediate locus of control of the cafeteria. How much money are you prepared to risk to follow your dream?

Personal threats arrive in the form of bad employees causing defamation, making it difficult to build a reputation in the community by the spreading of malicious rumours. Too many working hours would cause workers to experience burnout syndrome after a given amount of time (subject to individual's tolerance threshold).
Environmental - risks of market saturation, thereby witnessing customers disperse amongst other coffee shop businesses provides the need for reevaluation. Premier question to ask beforehand 'are their enough customers in the area?' It could be said that the only certainty is uncertainty.[110] Traffic disturbance from passing vehicles could also be a serious factor in a customer's decision.

Financial - retail costs may not be adding up thereby causing a lack of available resources, including insufficient starting capital. Having the ability to service debt when in lean times also

---

[110] Rubin & Weisberg (2003:251) *In An Uncertain World: Tough choices from Wall Street to Washington* – Random House

depends on gaining regular clientele, sponsors and support. Break-even volume would need to be attained as a given; Setting-up costs are huge, as are the regular costs of operation. Loans may be necessary to cover start-up costs – if so payback becomes expensive with interest, as do monthly rental charges.

Initiatives to cover threats could include a recognized and reputable equipment guarantee to save further expense from break-downs. Essentially the general public deserve good reasons why they should switch to Quasar Coffee Shop with maximum confidence, creating credibility with no threat attached.

Rationale for beliefs: Today's coffee market is huge, more so because of fair trade and the organic coffee generation. Retail outlets are able to support the growers and in doing so the system can be founded on a certain degree of trust. This therefore means that the whole operation can be performed to an optimum level by which customers can enjoy drinking the coffee in view of a fairer system. Quasar Coffee Shop would support fair trade/organic products.

Small businesses have a very welcome place in the community. Society relies on these enterprises to make a thriving local community. Looking around Hull, Beverley and York especially it could be said that small business represents the life-blood of these towns. With this in mind it could be said that a new coffee shop enterprise would be fully supported and welcomed with open arms into the marketplace arena.

Market research has a great responsibility in uncovering potential threats and opportunities, subsequently actions can be taken and decisions made according to findings. Where people know where they belong both opportunities and threats can be dealt with constructively, creatively, and progressively. To provide the best quality beverages, the tastiest sustenance, with the warmest most personable customer- friendly style would be an apparent aim for Quasar.

The Green Dragon

Financial projections[111]

Value proposition:– Local cafes stated start-up rates between £10k to £130k, therefore would be reasonable to assume a figure of £35k to start up.

Daily income:– Best scenario turnover = £3,000; Worst scenario turnover = £150. Based on 600 guests maximum, 85 guests minimum. Refer to customer base below.

Daily outgoing[112]:– Barista salary £5.75/hour. Friday staff covers 27 hours £155.25, Tuesday staff covers 34 hours £195.50 – average outgoing £175 plus overheads and contribution calculated/month.

Weekly income:– Same premise as above, best scenario = £21,000, worst scenario = £1,050 – rationale explained in Customer Base paragraph.

Weekly outgoing:– 220 hours amongst 6 staff calculates at £1265/week. Minimum rate for 24 hours £138 (William), to 45 hours maximum £258 (Bethany). Average outgoing £198/barista during a typical week.

Monthly income:- <£50,000 maximum, >£4,200 minimum. Premise as before.

Monthly outgoing:– Wages £5,060, Overheads £1,450, Contribution £2,500, Rent £1,200, Utilities £500, Product rejuvenation £10k – average outgoing £18k.

Monthly scenarios:- Best scenario (35k-20.7k = 14.3k) £14,300 profit, worst scenario (4.2k-12k= (8k)) £8,000 debt (and more). Likely turnover/month = £800 - £2,250.

Annual income:- From above scenarios profit range (30k) - £120k.

Annual expenditure:– Wages £60,720, Cost of sales £120k, Product costs 35% sales,   Food and drink cost approx 40%; 30%-35% labour cost; and a 20%-22% overheads cost, leaving a

---

[111] all projections based on existing prices and current budget available (k=£1,000)

[112] refer to appendix 3: example weekly staff schedule Quasar Coffee Shop March 2006.

percentage profit of between 5%-10%[113]. Rent £14,400, Utilities £6,000

Tradesmen paid at £25/hour: Plumbers £250/job, Decorators £350/job, Electrician £275/job, Joiners £420/job, Furniture removal/delivery £220/job, Marketing £75/1,000 flyers, Radio Broadcasting £free, Newspaper Advertising £20/month.

Inventory for furnishings: Armchairs £85/item, Sofa £260, Divan £180, Tables £15/item * 24, Chairs £12/item * 100, Bean bags £10 each, Art décor £30 -£350,

Fish in a tank £110, Plant life £180, (Taxidermy ◇£3,000), Entertainment podium £300, Stereo equipment £360, Coffee making technology £250, Crockery £320,

Tupperware £185, Cutlery £100, Kitchen Utensils £135, Cash register £125, Miscellaneous cleaning materials £220 : Proposed Totals 1610 + 6590 = £8,200.

Itemised costs for refreshments

Coffee beverages:- Latte small £1.10, regular £1.30, large £1.50, Cappuccino small £1.50, regular £1.75, large £1.95, Espresso £1.05, Americano small £1.05, regular £1.20, large £1.45, American dream small £1.50 Large £1.80, Decaffeinated small £1.05, regular £1.25, large £1.45, Selection of Fresh Roasted filter coffee Blue Mountain , Leonardo, Columbian Blend, Kenyan Decaf, Costa Rican – regular £1.50.

Coffee beans:- Vienna Roast £2.65/125g, Italian Continental £2.90/125g, French Roast £2.90/125g, Africa Kenya Peaberry £2.90/125g, SE Asia Java Jampit £3.95/125g, C&S America Peru El Guabo £2.90/125g, Colombian coffee beans £4.95/250g, Lincoln and York Espresso Beans £4.75/250g, Nescafe Decaffeinated Beans £2.65/125g, Italian beans £4.15/250g, Westminster beans £4.95/250g.

---

[113] http://search.epnet.com/login.aspx?direct=true&db=buh&an=9263243 Janet Harmer "Pull your socks up" Dec 2002/Jan 2003 Issue 42 p10, Business Source Premier

The Green Dragon

Chocolate/Malted beverages:- Mocha small £1.55, regular £1.80, large £2.15, Hot Chocolate small £1.20, regular £1.35, large £1.65 (plus supplements), Chocolate Expressos £1.60, Horlicks Malted small £1.10, regular £1.45, large £1.85.

Blended Green Teas: £1.20/mug eg Orange Pekoe, Peppermint, Lemon and Ginger, Liquorice, Camomile, Exotic Fruits et al, Regular tea £1.10/mug (Tetleys), Quality tea £1.35/mug (Earl Grey/Darjeeling/English Breakfast/Twinings)

Milk drinks:- regular glass £0.85 (Pasteurised, Semi-skimmed, UHT, Soya, Goats, Sterilised or Full fat), Milkshakes - strawberry, chocolate, banana, vanilla: Standard glass £1.85

Fruit juice/Soft drinks:- Orangina bottle £1.35, Freshly squeezed fruit juice small £0.95, large £1.30, Iced Macchiato regular £1.80, Smoothies regular size assorted ingredients available £2.15, Can of Pop £0.50, Large glass of Pop £1.20 Coca-Cola, Lemonade, Fanta, Ginger Ale, Appletise.

Food stuffs:- Soup and a bun £2.60, Salad (Caesar/Greek) £1.85, Homemade quiche and salad £3.50, Sandwich (bacon/sausage) £1.95, Full English Breakfast £3.15, Ham and Cheese toasty £1.50, Panini (various fillings and salad) £3.10, French Fries £0.89,   Bagels with cream cheese £0.88, Fresh fruit £0.32/piece, Tea and toast £1.60,
Muffins £1.40, Donuts £0.65, Scones £0.60, Slice of cake £1.20, Whole Gateau £15,
Assorted confectionery at £0.38/bar.

Customer base:– on a good day Quasar could experience up to 600 guests, and on a slow day at least 85 customers could visit to seek refreshment. Therefore, assuming the minimum purchase to be a small Café Latte, the minimum daily income would amount to £93.50 (1.10*85=93.50). Assuming a maximum lunchtime purchase to be quiche and salad, muffin, piece of fruit, and a smoothie, on a good day there is potential to make up to £1,842 (3.50 + 1.40 + 0.32 + 2.15 * 250 = 1,842). Likewise, a maximum breakfast purchase may include full English breakfast, tea and toast, with a large cappuccino, therefore (3.15 + 1.60 + 1.95 * 150 = 1,005) £1,005. An optimum day would see over £3,000 at Quasar Coffee Shop.

Research Methodology, findings and analysis

Quasar operates as a *sole trader*. The associated problem making the owner (myself) personally liable for *all* the debts of the business no matter how large. Baristas cost money! Six financial drivers of import include[114]: 1) cash available from daily clientele, 2) sales made encourage confidence in the business, 3) profit margins can be realized, in so doing Quasar receives consolidation, 4) margins of safety or break-even provide the structure necessary for orientation, 5) productivity represents the living business, 6) debtor or stock turnover exposes any weak points allowing for strengthening action.

In designing the questionnaire certain criteria would help enormously[115]. The art of asking questions can make the entire difference between success or failure, avoiding complex or ambiguous questions, keeping simple conversational language with no leading or loaded questions. No double-barrelled items. Assumptions should always be avoided unless substantial evidence is available to consolidate opinion. Burdensome questions that may toy the respondent's memory should also be avoided. On accounting for order bias, I arranged the sequence to begin with simple filter questions until the pivot q14 to elicit financial details (appendix 5 for questionnaire).

Collecting primary data from the selected respondents for this independent study meant the formation of a tailored questionnaire. Important considerations[116] would be timeframe (7 months), clarity of purpose of the study (Quasar Cafe), ensuring anonymity and confidentiality of the respondent, reinforce the importance of the respondent's participation by

---

[114] Burns P (2001:145-149)
[115] Zikmund W G (2003:ch15)
[116] Hair Bush Ortinau (2003:470)

acknowledging any reasons for non-completion of the survey, and demonstrating gratitude towards respondents for their time and insight.

Limitations came in the form of systematic error - the questions could always be made more specific. There has to be a limit within which to maintain inquiry. Respondent error by refusal and non-response, also response bias due to conflict of status/reputation, could cause defamation to occur, even deliberate falsification especially regarding company matters[117]. Unconscious misrepresentation often causes untoward outcomes without the speaker even realising.

Five stages of venture development could run as follows - Stage one would concern research and information collection. Stage two would be to assimilate this information and make some realistic projections from the existing facts. Stage three would involve the practical application of what theory is known into the reality of owning and operating a living business. Stage four would account for winning customers into your own business and ensuring loyalty to support the cause. Stage five would therefore be an appraisal of how well/successful is the business. Is Quasar liable to thrive and survive, or will we sink, swim and be forced to reevaluate?

Conclusions and recommendations

Strengths and Weaknesses related to starting-up the Quasar venture have been taken into consideration, notably having a passion for coffee, being able to create something unique and bringing excellence to the marketplace, whilst at the same time presenting a friendly disposition towards customers and staff alike. The main weakness would be lack of experience in professional ownership.

Opportunities and Threats have also been considered. Promotions within the coffee shop venture would enhance

---

[117] Zikmund W G (2003:174-189)

reputation and improve credibility with customers, such as the use of coffee cards where accumulated points can be redeemed for free food or drink. The most apparent challenges would be in being able to break-even and meet all costs whilst increasing the chances of making some profit on a regular basis. The huge growth in non-smoking coffee bars, non-smoking eating out experiences of all kinds over the past two decades suggests that people will continue to want to spend their money "out" somewhere[118].

Finances are variable, although a zone of activity can be painted, therefore the most valuable asset in running Quasar would be to take an objective view point and be fully
equipped to deal with situations as they occur. When the finances arrive you need to know how to deal with them, in this way lean times can be used constructively in preparation for better times.

Research for this independent study has occurred both via survey respondents in local coffee shops and useful theories from text books, e-journals, periodicals, word of mouth, and other sources. The major limitation on this project is the word limit. Quasar has a lot of potential for development, subsequent continuation with the project could ensure only that the quality of coffee improves for the guests by the time the bean arrives in hot liquid form in a Quasar's mug!

(Word Count 5,064)

---

[118]

http://proquest.umi.com/pqdweb?did=992707961&sid=2&Fmt=3&clientId=25727&RQT=309&VName=PQD Centaur Communications ltd "Smoking ban: what next for smoke-free pubs?" Marketing week Proquest London Feb 23 2006 p34

Bibliography/References

Books
Burns, P (2001) *Entrepreneurship and Small Business* – Palgrave
Hair Bush Ortinau (2003) *Marketing Research within a changing environment 2nd edition* : McGraw Hill Irwin
Hisrich R D & Peters M P (2002) *Entrepreneurship 5th International Edition* : McGraw-Hill Irwin
Ibbetson A OBE Pitman's *Common Commodities and industries – Tea from grower to consumer* 2nd edition : The Pitman Press Bath
Keable BB revised by Sanderson H S Pitman's *Common Commodities and industries – Coffee from grower to consumer* : The Pitman Press Bath
Timmons J A & Spinelli S (2003) *New Venture Creation – entrepreneurship for the 21st Century 6th International Edition* : McGraw Hill
Zikmund W G (2003) *Business Research Methods 7th edition* : Thomson South Western

World Wide Web
http://www.costa.co.uk/fairtrade/index.jsp
http://www.timhortons.com/en/about/index.html
http://starbucks.co.uk/en-GB/_About+Starbucks/
http://www.caffenero.com/CompanyInfo.asp?Section=Philosophy
http://www.caferouge.co.uk/aboutFrameset.html
http://search.epnet.com/login.aspx?direct=true&db=buh&an=9263243 Harmer, Janet (Dec 2002/Jan 2003) *"Pull your socks up"* Issue 42 p10, Business Source Premier EBSCO Host research database re Richard Shepherd restaurateur.
http://proquest.umi.com/pqdweb?did=992707961&sid=2&Fmt=3&clientId=25727&RQT=309&VName=PQD Centaur Communications ltd "Smoking ban: what next for smoke-free pubs?" Marketing week Proquest London Feb 23 2006 p34

Newspapers & Journals

Appendix 1[119]

Initiatives demonstrated by Costa Coffee

Gino Amasanti comments: "In order to serve the best coffee in our authentic Italian style, Costa owns the entire coffee production process from bean to cup including sourcing, roasting and testing the beans. This move means we have the same control over our fairtrade coffee and helps to showcase its quality and close the gap between coffee growers and coffee lovers on the high street".

Harriet Lamb, Director, Fairtrade Foundation: "Costa Coffee were one of the first company's to offer the choice of fairtrade certified coffee and tea and we raise our cups to celebrate this furthering of their commitment to fairtrade. This is good news for Costa's customers who want fairtrade and of course good news for the coffee farmers".

As pioneers of café culture in the UK, Costa inspired the creation of popular and convenient concessions stores in locations such as Waterstones and Ottakars bookstores, and BAA outlets. A welcome respite for shoppers to relax, unwind and enjoy a revitalising cup of coffee crafted the Italian way.

---

[119]

http://proquest.umi.com/pqdweb?did=996799081&sid=2&Fmt=3&clientId=25727&RQT=309&VName=PQD "What's under your froth? Drinking with a conscience as Costa launches its own blend of fair trade coffee" Proquest New York March 03 2006 PR Newswire Europe including UK Disclose

Appendix 2[120] Managerial approach at Quasar very much focuses on stage 3.

Classification of Moral Judgement into Stages of Development

Stage	Orientation	Theme
1	Punishment and obedience	Morality of obedience
2	Instrumental relativism	Simple exchange
3	Interpersonal concordance	Reciprocal role taking
4	Law and order	Formal justice
5	Legitimate social contact	Procedural justice
6	Universal ethical principle	Individual conscience

Exhibit 10 adapted from Kohlberg (1967)

Appendix 3 Example weekly staff schedule at Quasar Coffee Shop March 2006

	Mon	Tue	Wed	Thu	Fri	Sat	Sun	Hours
Donna		13:00 – 23:00	14:30 – 20:00	15:00 – 23:00	13:00 – 19:30		13:00 – 20:00	37
Steve	13:00 – 23:00		14:00 – 23:00	13:00 – 23:00		13:00 – 20:00		36
Beth	13:00 – 23:00	07:00 – 13:45		07:00 – 13:15		08:00 – 20:00	08:00 – 20:00	45
Anna	07:00 – 15:00		07:00 – 15:00		07:00 – 13:00	14:00 – 20:00	14:00 – 20:00	34

---

[120] Timmons & Spirelli (2003:335) New Venture Creation 6th International ed - McGraw Hill

Wills		07:00 – 15:00		07:00 – 15:00	15:00 – 23:00			24
Jamie	07:00 – 13:00	14:00 – 23:00	07:00 – 14:30		07:00 – 14:30	08:00 – 14:30	08:30 – 14:30	45
Hours	34	34	29	32	27	31.5	31	**220**

Shifts are flexible and baristas on rotation each week. 45 hours is considered maximum for any one employee, and 16 hours minimum. Wages (£5.75/hour) are adjustable depending on employee performance.

Appendix 4[121]
Coffee shops visited (in alphabetical order):-
- Bain Café - Lincoln Campus, Hull University
- Betty's Café Tea Rooms – St Helens Square, York
- Café Ha Ha – New Street, York
- Café Nero – Market Place, Beverley
- Café Nero – Davygate, York
- Café Rouge – Low Petergate, York
- Café One – Newland Avenue, Hull
- Café Uno – Clifford Street, York
- Continental Café Bar - Hull University Student Union
- Fudge Café/Restaurant – Princes Avenue, Hull
- Gingers – Swabys Yard, Beverley
- Helmsley Arts Centre Coffee Shop
- Latitude café/restaurant - Newland Avenue, Hull
- Lemon Tree café - York City Railway Station
- Pavement Café – New Street, York
- Planet Coffee – Newland Avenue, Hull
- Relax Coffee Shop – Newland Avenue, Hull
- Starbucks - Borders Bookstore, Davygate, York

---

[121] all my completed coffee shop questionnaires available on request

The Green Dragon

- Starbucks - Coppergate, York
- Tesco Coffee shop - Beverley
- The Sun Café - Cottingham Road, Hull
- Turpins Coffee House – Butcher Row, Beverley
- Victor J's Café/Bar – Finkle Street, York
- Zest Café/Restaurant – Newland Avenue, Hull

Appendix 5 *Sample Questionnaire*

1) What is the name of the coffee shop?
....
....

2) Which varieties of coffee do you sell to drink here?
....
....
....

3) Where do you get your coffee from? (Which country/ies)
....
....
....

4) What other beverages do you offer here besides coffee?
....
....
....
....

5) Is it an independent branch or part of a chain?
....
....

6) What is the seating capacity of your coffee shop?
....
....

7) How many employees work for the business? (at this branch? entire chain?)

....
....
....
....

8) For how long has this coffee shop been operating?
....
....
....

9) How many customers typically visit here on a – good/average/bad – day?
....
....
....
....

10) What are your regular opening hours?
....
....
....
....

11) What skills are most useful in running your coffee shop business?
....
....
....
....
....
....
....

12) Which customer needs are taken into account within the café? (eg décor, location, products, service, prices, promotions, entertainments) and how would you describe them (contemporary/traditional/archaic)?

The Green Dragon

....
....
....
....
....
....
....
....
....
....
....
....
....

13) How is the management structure organised here?
....
....
....
....
.
....
....
....
....

14) Are you operating with a view to expand, or with a view to maximise business in this particular branch alone?
....
....
....

15) Would you itemise, and price, a selection of your products please?
....
....
....
....
....
....

16) How much did it cost to open this branch initially?

....
....

17) What would be the typical monthly cost and profit to the business?

....
....
....
....

18) What would be the typical annual cost and profit to the business?

....
....
....
....
....
....

19) What risks would need to be accounted for on starting a small business operation such as with an independent branch coffee shop?

....
....
....
....
....
....
....
....
....

20) How do you view the competition…ie how do you stay one step ahead?

....
....
....

The Green Dragon

....
....
....
....
....
......

Thankyou very much for your time and for completing this questionnaire!

THIS CONCLUDES THE GREEN DRAGON

Lightning Source UK Ltd.
Milton Keynes UK
UKHW041611140520
363228UK00001B/65

9 781849 915250